Probiotic Rescue

■ ■ ■ ■ ■ ■ ■

Probiotic Rescue

How You Can Use Probiotics to Fight Cholesterol,
Cancer, Superbugs, Digestive Complaints and More

■ ■ ■ ■ ■ ■ ■

ALLISON TANNIS, MSc., RHN

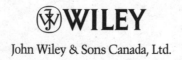

John Wiley & Sons Canada, Ltd.

Library and Archives Canada Cataloguing in Publication Data

Tannis, Allison
    Probiotic rescue: how you can use probiotics to fight cholesterol, cancer superbugs, digestive complaints and more / Allison Tannis.

Includes bibliographical references and index.
ISBN 978-0-470-15475-5

    1. Probiotics—Popular works. I. Title.

RM666.P835T35 2008   615'.329   C2008-900610-0

Production Credits
Cover and interior text design: Tegan Wallace
Typesetter: Thomson Digital
Printer: Friesens

John Wiley & Sons Canada, Ltd.
6045 Freemont Blvd.
Mississauga, Ontario
L5R 4J3

This book is printed with biodegradable vegetable-based inks. Text pages are printed on 551b 100% PCW Hibulk, Natural by Friesens Corp., an FSC certified printer.

Printed in Canada

1 2 3 4 5 FP 12 11 10 09 08

For Mimi — a woman who inspires us all to make a difference

Table of Contents

■ ■ ■ ■ ■ ■ ■

PART III: Safety, Products and the Future of Probiotics

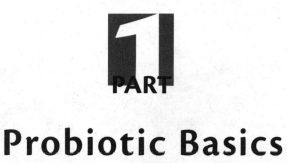

Probiotic Basics

chapter

1

Probiotics 101

A MICROSCOPIC VIEW OF THIS CHAPTER

- Both good and bad microbes live in your body.
- Bad microbes can cause illness.
- Probiotics are good microbes that live in your body.
- Probiotics inhibit the growth of bad microbes.
- Probiotics assist with digestion, nutrient absorption and vitamin production.
- Probiotics affect the health of the immune system.
- Different probiotics have different effects on your health.
- The key to a healthy microflora is to maintain a healthy population of a diversity of good microorganisms.

■ ■ ■ ■ ■ ■ ■

If you tend to be squeamish you may not want to know that your intestinal tract is home to one hundred trillion (10^{14}) **microorganisms**. Microorganisms are bacteria and yeasts that are not visible to the human eye. In fact, microorganisms are all around you. They are in the water you drink, the food you eat and the air you breathe. Don't worry—about 95% of microorganisms are good for you. Microorganisms, sometimes called **microbes**, include bacteria, viruses, fungi, yeasts, algae and protozoa.

The microorganisms that live in your intestines make up what is called the intestinal **microflora**. The intestinal microflora is made up of many types of bacteria, fungi and yeast. Knowing that bacteria are

In your body there are more microbes than human cells. the chief cause of infectious diseases in humans, it can be hard to imagine that they also play a beneficial role in your body.

In your body, there are over 400 different species of microbes, living in symbiosis with you—their host. Bacteria can be found in your mouth, stomach, intestines and **urogenital** tract. Some bacteria found in your body are known to be beneficial to human health and are called **probiotics**. Meanwhile, the other bacteria in your body, which are harmful, are called **pathogenic** bacteria. Depending on the type of bacteria, there is a different effect on the body; bacteria can have healthy, e.g., immune-boosting, benefits or cause **toxicological** (poisoning) harm to the body. A careful balance is necessary for health. The growth of harmful microbes in your body can result in disease.

The 400 species of microbes living in your body are fighting for space. They want to live, thrive and reproduce in your intestinal tract, an environment that offers the ideal temperature, humidity and food sources. Who wins the battle for your intestinal tract? Your intestinal tract is a complex community of microbes. Do you have the right microbes in you?

Bacterial Basics

Bacteria are unicellular, e.g., one-cell, and may have spherical, rod-like or curved bodies. Bacteria are very small. On average, bacteria are about one micrometer long and half a micrometer in diameter. The bacteria cell is surrounded by a **membrane** that regulates the flow of materials in and out. Some species of bacteria are surrounded by a capsule which has many functions, including protecting the bacteria from drying. Many species of bacteria swim by means of flagella, hair-like structures whose whip-like lashing provides movement. *NOTE:* When applied to bacteria, the term "growth" refers to an increase in the size of a population rather than an increase in the size of an individual microorganism.

BAD AND GOOD MICROBES

Similar to many childhood tales, the intestinal tract is an ongoing battle between good and evil. There are two types of microbes in your body: the bad and the good. Bad microbes live in your intestines and normally do not cause any disease-like symptoms. Fungi, yeasts and bacteria all live in the body and can be classified as bad microbes. Two examples of bad microbes commonly found in the human body are the bacteria E. *coli* and the yeast *Candida albicans*. What favors the growth of these bad microbes? Bad microbes flourish in an **alkaline** environment. Many of them produce ammonia to change the pH of the intestinal tract to be more alkaline and thus enhance their ability to survive and flourish. Stress and diet can also influence the presence of these microbes. Keeping these bad microbes in control is vital to the body's health.

There are also good microbes found in the body, called **probiotics**. Probiotics have a positive impact on the body's health. They prefer a more acidic intestinal environment. Many of the probiotics are called **lactic acid bacteria**. They can secrete lactic acid into their environment, making it more acidic and thus more hospitable to them. Stress and diet can reduce the number of probiotics in the intestinal tract. Luckily, as most childhood tales of good versus evil end in a positive light, so does this story. In a healthy body the majority of the microflora in the intestines is good bacteria, also known as probiotics.

PROBIOTICS

What is a probiotic? The term *probiotic* originates from the ancient Greek words *pro* and *biotica*, meaning "for life." In 2001, an Expert Consultation meeting arranged by the World Health Organization and the Food and Agriculture Organization of the United Nations created a now widely accepted definition for probiotics. They define the term probiotic as:

> *live microorganisms which when administered in adequate amounts confer a health benefit on the host.*

Medically, probiotic is defined as microorganisms that positively affect the health of our body when administered in adequate amounts.

A probiotic offers a health benefit to the host. What are these health benefits? First, let us consider the microflora as a whole. The intestinal microflora has the metabolic activity potential equal to that of the liver, the most active organ in the body! As such, the microflora is sometimes referred to as the "forgotten organ." Be kind to your intestinal microbes as they contribute greatly to your metabolism.

| *The intestinal microflora has the metabolic activity potential equal to that of the liver.*

Of all the species in the microflora, those designated as probiotics are of most importance to your body's health. Probiotics affect many aspects of the body including nutrient digestion and absorption, immunity and much more. Probiotics aid digestion by completing the breakdown of food that was not fully digested. A good example is the ability of certain strains of probiotics to help with the digestion of lactose in the small intestine. As well, probiotics strains found in the colon help with digestion of some forms of fiber. Probiotics also produce vitamins, including the particularly important B vitamins, which play a key role in energy metabolism.

Probiotics have other roles in promoting health in your body. They can inhibit the ability of bad microbes to grow in the intestines. This can help prevent illness and disease. Many strains of probiotics are lactic acid bacteria. This means they are capable of releasing lactic acid into the environment. By producing lactic acid, certain probiotics can lower the pH of the intestinal tract, making the environment unfriendly to bad microbes and thus reducing the growth of bad microbes that can cause illness. Certain probiotics can also excrete **antimicrobial** substances. Antimicrobials kill pathogenic microbes. Probiotics also prevent the growth of bad microbes by competing for nutrients and receptor sites in the intestinal tract. In fact, there are a number of mechanisms by which probiotics inhibit the **colonization** of pathogenic microbes in the intestinal tract, many of which will be discussed in Chapter 3.

Perhaps the greatest health benefit that probiotics offer is the promotion of a healthy immune system. The intestines are lined with cells called **epithelial** cells. These are the same cells that make up your skin. Epithelial cells are specially designed to help the body carefully interact with its environment. When you eat food it contains a lot of foreign things, including bacteria, pesticides and preservatives which interact with the epithelial cells that line the intestinal tract. This interaction can be negative or positive. If the pesticide you ate interacts with your intestinal epithelial cells and the body decides it is a foreign invader an immune reaction will occur in an attempt to rid the body of this invader. This is a negative interaction. When probiotics attach to receptor sites on the epithelial lining of the intestinal wall, the interaction is positive. Probiotics send communications to nearby immune cells. This has positive effects on the immune system that can affect the entire body. Clinical and population studies have shown this interaction between microbes in our intestinal tract, the epithelial cells and eventually the immune cells to be beneficial in the body. In fact, the ability of microbes to positively affect the immune system is known to help prevent illness and to be helpful in the treatment of certain allergic, inflammatory and chronic diseases.

In addition, probiotics play a key role in the maturation of the immune system. The intestinal tract is sterile at birth but eventually hosts 10^{14} **CFU**/mL (CFU stands for colony-forming units, a measurement of how many living groups of probiotics are present) of microbes representing between 400 and 500 species. The intestinal microflora develops gradually as we age and is influenced by factors including our mother's microflora and our diet, use of antibiotics, stress, hygiene, environment and possibly genetics. We know that probiotics play an important role in the maturation of the immune system from scientific studies on a germ-free **animal model**. In a germ-free animal, there are no microbes living in the intestinal tract. In these animals, the lack of microbes was associated with a greatly underdeveloped immune system. In other words, if there are no microbes in an intestinal tract, the immune system does not develop fully. Probiotics are very important to your immune health.

Colony-forming unit (CFU) is a measure of microbes. Unlike in direct microscopic counts where all cells, dead and living, are counted, CFU measures only living cells. The theory behind the CFU technique is that a single bacteria can grow and become a colony, via binary fission. Binary fission is the form of reproduction by microbes in which one cell divides into two cells. Each colony that forms is clearly different from each other, making it easy to count each colony as one CFU.

Probiotics also help maintain a healthy gastrointestinal tract. Commonly known for their ability to improve constipation, probiotics can also alleviate some forms of diarrhea and promote general wellness of the lining of the gastrointestinal tract. Digestive diseases are on the rise. According to the National Digestive Disease Information Clearinghouse (NDDIC), digestive disease, including irritable bowel disease syndrome and ulcers, affect between 60 and 70 million people in the United States alone. In Canada, diarrhea alone accounts for approximately 150,000 sick days per year with an estimated cost of $22 million to the health care system. Poor eating habits, eating lots of highly processed foods, over-consumption of food and stress are contributing factors to this rise in digestive diseases. You may notice that these factors are very similar to those affecting the number of probiotics in your intestinal tract. It is likely that probiotics play a role in these digestive ailments. Research into the positive effects of probiotics on diarrhea, irritable bowel disease, ulcerative colitis, pouchitis and Crohn's disease offers promise as a method to relieve some of the burden these diseases place on society.

There are many health benefits offered by probiotics to the host: improved digestion, immunity and health. However, it is important to realize that each probiotic species is different and thus has different abilities and effects on human health. Each probiotic species has its own health effects. As such, it is important to learn which probiotic has which health effect. To fully understand the potential of probiotics for health, we need to discover in which regions they live in the body, what they do and how they affect the human body.

PROBIOTICS IN THE GASTROINTESTINAL TRACT

The gastrointestinal tract starts in your mouth, travels through the stomach, intestines and ends at the anus. In each section of the gastrointestinal tract, you will find different types and quantities of microbes. All in all, the average adult carries about four pounds of microbes in their intestinal tract.

In the mouth, there are many types of microbes. Almost 500 bacterial strains have been identified in this oral pocket. Contrary to the esophagus where there are no microbes, the stomach is host to one hundred thousand (10^8 CFU/mL) microbes. Streptococcus, Lactobacillus, *Candida albicans* and *Helicobacter pylori* are common microbes found in the stomach.

The first part of the small intestine is called the **duodenum**. About 5 centimeters down the duodenum you'll find the location where the **pancreas** secretes bile salts into the intestinal tract. The pancreas is responsible for creating the enzymes that break down the food you eat into small pieces that the body can absorb. The bile salts from the pancreas have a basic pH. Their presence drastically changes the pH of the intestines from the very acidic pH of the stomach to a more neutral pH. The stomach and small intestine have strong acidic and basic environments, and a relatively swift flow of materials. As such, the stomach and small intestine have relatively low concentrations of microflora as this is a difficult environment to live in. To humans, it would be like living in an environment with high winds and drastic changes in temperature from very hot to very cold.

The duodenum is host to 10,000 to 100,000 (10^4 to 10^5 CFU/mL) microbes. The microbial species found here are from the bacterial families Streptococcus and Lactobacillus, as well as Bacterioides and the yeast *Candida albicans*. In the **jejunum**, the second section of the small intestine, there are even more microbes present. About one million to 100 millon (10^5 to 10^7 CFU/mL) of microbes, including species from the genus Streptococcus. Lactobacillus, the yeast *Candida albicans* and Bacteroides are also present here. The final section of the small intestine is the **ileum**, where there are 100 million to one billion (10^6 to 10^9 CFU/mL) of microbes including species from the genera Lactobacilli, Enterococci, Bacteroides, Veillonella, Clostridium and Enterobacteria.

In the **colon** we find the greatest concentration of microflora; about 10^{10} to 10^{11} CFU/mL. The colon microflora is made up of Bacteroides, Bifidobacterium, Clostridium, Ruminococcus, Peptostreptococcus, Fusobacterium, Eubacterium, Bacillus, Streptococci and Enterococci. In fact, there are about 1.5 kilograms of microbes present in the colon.

MICROFLORA DIVERSITY

Just as each of us has unique fingerprints, we also have a unique mix of intestinal microbes. The makeup of your intestinal microflora began

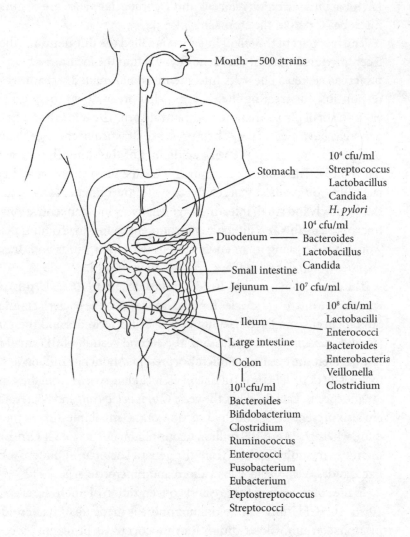

Mouth — 500 strains

Stomach —
10^4 cfu/ml
Streptococcus
Lactobacillus
Candida
H. pylori

Duodenum —
10^4 cfu/ml
Bacteroides
Lactobacillus
Candida

Small intestine

Jejunum — 10^7 cfu/ml

Ileum
10^8 cfu/ml
Lactobacilli
Enterococci
Bacteroides
Enterobacteria
Veillonella
Clostridium

Large intestine

Colon

10^{11} cfu/ml
Bacteroides
Bifidobacterium
Clostridium
Ruminococcus
Enterococci
Fusobacterium
Eubacterium
Peptostreptococcus
Streptococci

Figure 1-1: Diagram of the Intestinal Tract Illustrating Common Microbes Present in Each Section.

to take shape at birth. Then depending on whether you were breast or bottle fed, different types of microbes were added. Over time, your individual diet, environment and lifestyle choices have shaped and personalized your microflora.

The key to a healthy microflora in your body is to maintain a large number of good microbes in your digestive tract. An overwhelming balance of good over bad bacteria is important. Several factors can negatively affect this balance: these include aging, depressed immunity, digestive tract infections, environmental pollution, poor diet, stress and diarrhea. As well, the use of antibiotics affects your natural microflora. We live in a world filled with **antibiotic** and **antibacterial** products. We have become bacteria-phobic. The focus has been on fighting "bad" bacteria. The result is a loss of not just bad bacteria but good bacteria, including probiotics. Without probiotics we can become ill.

The normal ratio of probiotics to harmful microbes should be approximately 85% to 15%. This balance of good to bad can be disrupted by stress, a poor diet or infection by a bad microbe. If there is an overgrowth of bad microbes (pathogens) in your body, antibiotics may be necessary to regain balance. For example, strep throat can be caused by an overgrowth of a nasty bacteria, which, if not treated with antibiotics, runs the risk of developing into a serious infection. Antibiotics might seem like a good idea, but using them further disrupts your microflora. Antibiotics not only destroy the bad bacteria, which are causing you to be sick, but they also destroy good bacteria living in the digestive tract. Both antibiotics and antibacterial products can cause an imbalance in our body's microflora by reducing the number of probiotics. When the composition of the intestinal microflora is disrupted, there can be negative effects on the health of the body. As such, it may be necessary to re-establish your body's probiotic population. How can you do this? Simple—ingest probiotics. The intestinal microflora can be replenished and restored to its healthy strength and balance by taking probiotic supplements and eating probiotic-enriched foods.Yogurt, supplements and many foods offer you an easy source of probiotics to help regain the balance. **Prebiotics** can also help encourage the growth of probiotics in your body. Prebiotics are the food that probiotics eat. Prebiotics are carbohydrates that your body can not digest, so they are left for the probiotics to enjoy. Chapter 5 is dedicated to prebiotics.

It is now obvious that maintaining a sufficient population of probiotics in your intestinal tract is important to your health. But, why

> **Prebiotics**
>
> Prebiotics are nondigestible food ingredients that stimulate the growth and health of good bacteria in the colon and thus improve host health. Prebiotics include inulin, which is in onions, chichory root and dandelions; oligosaccharides, which is in artichokes, leeks and asparagus; beta-glucan, which is in seaweed, oats and barley; pectin, which is in apples and apricots and resistant starch, which is in raw bananas, potatoes and beans. Prebiotics are present in our daily diets; however, in very low amounts in the Western diet. See Chapter 5 for more on prebiotics.

do you need to host over 400 different species of microbes in your intestines? The diversity is needed as each species of probiotic has its own unique set of health benefits. One species may only offer two health benefits, while another species may offer two completely different health benefits. We need a variety of species to ensure we get the whole gamut of health benefits available. Also, probiotics can work **synergistically**, i.e., enhance the effect of each other, to offer an increased level of health to you. Probiotic health benefits include aiding in proper digestion; inhibiting pathogenic microbes; promoting a healthy immune system; and helping with some vitamin production. As such, having a diversity of probiotics in your intestines means you can maximize the likelihood of getting the entire, wide array of health benefits that probiotics have to offer.

SUMMARY

The human intestinal tract is host to many species of microbes, some of which are bad, others good. The good bacteria are called *probiotics*. Probiotics are key to a healthy body. Probiotics help with digestion, affect the health of the immune system, inhibit bad microbes living in the intestine and protect the intestinal lining from infection of more bad microbes. Different probiotics have different health benefits. The key to good health is to maintain a large, diverse number of probiotics in the body.

chapter
2

A History of Probiotics

A Microscopic View of This Chapter

- The idea of probiotics has existed for centuries.
- Probiotics were discovered at the end of the 19th century.
- Probiotics have healthy benefits.
- The makeup of microbes in your body changes with age.
- Recently, probiotic research has exploded and new discoveries happen frequently.
- Today probiotics are used around the world and new products are prevalent.
- The original source of probiotics varies.

■ ■ ■ ■ ■ ■ ■

Microbes, such as bacteria, existed long before humans evolved. These little organisms can be found on the tops of mountains, the bottom of the deepest oceans, in the intestines of animals and even in the frozen rocks and ice of Antarctica. Human history has been shaped by our interactions with microbes. Cholera, small pox and the plague are examples of how microbes have put humans at their mercy. However, these small creatures can also be as much of a blessing as a problem.

History is full of claims that living microbes in food, particularly lactic acid bacteria, can improve health. Remember that many probiotics are lactic acid bacteria. People have eaten fermented milk products which contain lactic acid bacteria since prebiblical times. In the Bible and the sacred books of Hinduism there are mentions of cultured dairy products being eaten. Other cultured dairy products, such as kefir and koumiss, originated many centuries ago. Kefir, derived from the Turkish word *keif*, which loosely translated means "good feeling," originated in the northern Caucasus mountains in Russia. Koumiss, a fermented alcoholic beverage prepared from milk, was known to the Scythians (7th century BC), according to the famous Greek historian, Herodotus. Today, in the same area of the world, which is now referred to as Siberia, fermented milk products are a staple in the diet.

The first scientist to identify a healthy bacteria, which is now classified as a probiotic, was Louis Pasteur, a French scientist. Pasteur identified Lactobacillus in the 1850s. This bacteria was found to occur naturally in yogurt and improved the health of people who ate it.

Discovery: Bacteria Can Help You

In the early 1900s, a predecessor of Pasteur's, Russian immunologist Dr. Eli Metchnikoff, suggested that a synergistic interaction exists between bacteria and their host. Metchnikoff noted the longevity of Bulgarian peasants who ate a lot of yogurt. He proposed that a link existed between better health and longer life and the consumption of lactic acid bacteria (probiotics) delivered to the intestine via yogurt. Dr. Metchnikoff's subsequent work on cellular immunity won him the Nobel prize in 1908.

Meanwhile, around 1900, Dr. Henry Tissier discovered Bifidobacteria. Tissier recommended the administration of Bifidobacteria to infants suffering from diarrhea, claiming that Bifidobacteria gets rid of the pathogenic bacteria that cause the disease. He also showed that Bifidobacteria were predominant in the gut flora of breast-fed infants.

Research in the area of probiotics was slow for many years after this groundbreaking discovery. However, researchers were able to uncover a better understanding of the relationship between probiotics and the human intestinal tract.

Discovery: Probiotics Prevent Disease

In the 1950s, scientific research in probiotics had a renewed interest. It was a group of scientists led by Freter, Collins, Carter and Bohnohoff who broadened our understanding of probiotics. They discovered that intestinal microflora helps an animal be resistant to disease. They discovered that mice that were given oral antibiotics, which kill all bacteria, including probiotics, were more susceptible to infection. As well, animals with microflora in their intestines had a better chance of survival than those with none. Their research offered more proof that good microflora (probiotics) offers protection from infections.

The term *probiotic* was not actually coined until the 1960s. Lilly and Stillwell first defined probiotics as "substances produced by microorganisms which promote the growth of other microorganisms." In 1974, Parker elaborated on the definition of *probiotic* to also include, "organisms and substances which contribute to intestinal microbial balance."

Discovery: Microflora Changes as We Age

In 1978, Dr. Tomotari Mitsuoka, a Japanese scientist, wrote *Intestinal Flora and Health*, still one of the main references in the study of lactic acid bacteria today. Mitsuoka illustrated how the composition of intestinal flora changes during a lifetime. He also demonstrated how amounts of

---

Definition of Probiotic

In October, 2001, an Expert Consultation meeting convened by the Food & Agriculture Organization (FAO) and World Health Organization (WHO) defined probiotic as "live microorganisms which when administered in adequate amounts confer a health benefit on the host." This definition has the following characteristics:

- Probiotics must deliver a measured physiological benefit, substantiated by studies conducted in the target host.
- Probiotics need not be restricted to food applications or oral delivery.
- A definition of probiotics should not limit the mechanism of action.
- Probiotics must be alive.

Although it was recognized that dead cells may have health benefits, the consultants suggested that a different term be used for dead cells to reflect to the consumer that probiotics are alive.

Bifidobacteria in the intestines decrease with age, increasing our risk of colon disease. His work supported the theory that the oral administration of probiotics, including Bifidobacteria, improves intestinal flora balance and helps prevent the development of lower bowel conditions.

More Discoveries Every Day

Thanks to these forefathers of probiotic research, today many potential health benefits of probiotics are being studied. Lactic acid bacteria play a key role in restoring and maintaining intestinal flora balance and enhancing immune system functions. Recent research is investigating lactic acid bacteria's potential **hypocholesterolemic** effects (lowers blood cholesterol levels), use as a treatment for urogential and vaginal diseases, as well as their role in colon cancer prevention and asthma. Plus, probiotics are being studied for their potential role in heart disease, oral health, prevention of the cold and flu, HIV-associated diarrhea, treatment of superbugs and much more. Researchers are also discovering more bacteria and yeasts that demonstrate probiotic effects and are showing promise as future therapies for diseases in humans.

From the Laboratory to Your Plate

The ability to take this research knowledge and transform it into easy, at-home therapies is what makes probiotics such a fascinating area. The hard work of these early researchers was first applied to products by the Yakult Company of Japan in the 1930s. Yakult Company introduced a fermented milk product that contained a probiotic culture. Today, Yakult milk product can be found in many countries around the world, including Australia, Europe and Taiwan. In Japan, one can find dozens of probiotic products on supermarket shelves, ranging from fortified milks to candy containing Lactobacilli and Bifidobacterium strains. In Chapter 18, we'll take a closer look at some of these products available on supermarket shelves.

The probiotic food trend is evident around the world. Most popular in Japan, probiotics are consumed to a lesser degree in Europe. The use of probiotic supplements in Europe is a booming segment of the supplement market. In fact, market data shows that probiotic drinks made up 30% of the functional food market in Europe just after the turn of the century. In Europe, the dairy sector is the most developed segment of the probiotic market. Fermented milks, probiotic drinks and yogurts are sold in convenient "daily dose" formats. These are the most widely used formats in Europe. However, consumer acceptance of probiotic products varies greatly across the region. For example, Scandinavian and Northern European countries that have a long tradition of eating fermented dairy products have the highest acceptance of probiotics. Other regions in Europe are slower to come on board. North America is also slowly joining in the probiotic movement.

North Americans are less accepting of probiotics than Europeans. An interesting difference is that North Americans are more willing to take a supplement than their European counterparts. This may explain the popularity of probiotic supplements despite the relatively low number of probiotic foods available in North America versus other global regions. However, a change is occurring as can be seen by the influx of probiotic foods in the North American market since the turn of the century. Probiotic yogurts entered the mainstream North American supermarket aisles early in the 21st century. Probiotic milks and cheeses slowly followed suit. The supermarket landscape in North America changed quickly as major probiotic manufacturers were teaming up with large U. S. dairy and food companies to produce more probiotic functional foods such as smoothies, candy, cereals and other fortified food and beverage items. This boom in innovative probiotic products in North America can also be seen around the world. Advances in probiotic research are likely fueling this growing interest in probiotics by the public. The boom in probiotics is not just latest health food flavor of the month—probiotics are supported by strong evidence that they support good health. They have been referred to as the next essential fatty acids (omega-3s) or the new vitamins. Probiotics are more than just the latest new cheese or yogurt, they are the next step in nutritional wellness.

WHERE DO PROBIOTICS COME FROM?

Where do all of these species of probiotics come from? Most of today's lactic acid bacteria strains used in probiotic supplements were isolated approximately 20 years ago from human, dairy and vegetal origins. It is these same strains that are found in the probiotic foods and supplements on the supermarket shelves today. Research conducted over two decades ago is relevant today, as the bacteria strains are the same. The same strains that were isolated 20 years ago and used in initial research studies are the same strains used in research today.

How did researchers isolate the probiotic strains? Research labs and universities used a three-phase method to select these strains.

- **Phase 1.** The Mother-strain or original probiotics is isolated using a process called *colony selection process*. Then, the strain is purified and identified. Researchers achieve this by a testing method called *Analytical Profile Identification*.
- **Phase 2.** The researchers look for the characterisitics of the probiotic strain such as its ability to survive and reproduce. These two characteristics are important if a probiotic is to surivive on the supermarket shelf and be able to reproduce in your intestines. Researchers can then determine what production methods should be used to maximize bacterial growth.
- **Phase 3.** Researchers discover the characteristics of the probiotic strain. Different tests define the exact characteristics of the strain. These characteristics include the probiotic strain's ability to fight bad microbes, produce enzymes that promote nutrient absorption and vitamin production and more. By identifying the characteristics of the strain, researchers can select the best probiotic for your health. In other words, all of this detailed work by scientists ensures that the probiotic strains found in today's products are those that offer us the best health benefit.

Today, probiotic manufacturers can offer consumers around the world safe and effective dosages of probiotics thanks to the long hours spent in laboratories by our scientific predecessors. Every day, researchers gain a greater understanding of the mechanisms of probiotics. However, it will likely take many decades more before the specific health benefits of each probiotic strain is fully understood. Until that time we can focus on what we do know: the use of a diversity of probiotic strains supports your health by boosting your immune system, improving your ability to uptake nutrients and helping to prevent and treat some disease conditions.

SUMMARY

Probiotics were discovered before the turn of the 20th century; however, research was slow in this field for the next hundred years. Over this time researchers discovered that probiotics can prevent disease and that a person's microflora changes with age. The term *probiotic* was first introduced in the 1960s, but a firm definition was not created until 2001. Today, new discoveries about probiotics are emerging at a rapid pace. New technology and growing interest by consumers is fueling this probiotic movement. On the market, dairy-based probiotics have been in existence in Japan for many years and are popular in Europe. North America is quickly increasing its interest in probiotics. The global interest in probiotics has resulted in a surge of innovative foods that contain probiotics. Researchers are linking probiotics with a wide array of health benefits and the number of disease conditions they are thought to benefit continues to grow.

3

How Probiotics Work: Probiotics' Mechanism of Action

A MICROSCOPIC VIEW OF THIS CHAPTER

- Inside your body is a war between good and bad microbes.
- Probiotics have many mechanisms of action.
- Probiotics prevent bad microbes from growing and causing disease.
- Bad microbes are inhibited by probiotics competing for receptor sites, masking sites and making the environment acidic.
- Probiotics produce enzymes that promote health.
- Probiotics produce antimicrobials that kill bad microbes.
- Probiotics support the health of cells that line the intestines.
- Probiotics work synergistically.
- Probiotics positively affect the immune system.
- Candida, *E. coli, H. pylori* and Salmonella can all be inhibited by probiotics.

■ ■ ■ ■ ■ ■ ■

A war is waging. The battles have commenced. Inside your body lie miles of intestines, bunched, curled and crammed into your abdomen. This is the battle ground of a life-long war—a war between good and evil. If only microbes were a more glamorous topic, this epic war would be the next blockbuster hit in Hollywood, but we are not likely to soon see Brad Pitt on the big screen, depicting this bacterial intestinal war.

Despite the lack of glamour and glitz, the war in your intestines between good and bad microbes is perhaps the most important war you'll ever learn of. Let's first look at why your intestines are exposed to incoming microbes. The intestines are exposed to almost everything in your environment. Food enters the body and brings along with it tons of chemicals, pollutants, dirt and microbes. As such, your intestines are one of the most important gatekeepers to your body. Entrance will only be granted to those worthy of entry. Like a castle wall in medieval times, your intestinal lining has a dangerous and important job. Invaders can charge the castle at any hour. As such, your intestines need to be armed with valiant, strong knights—and the more, the better.

Who is worthy of being a knight in your intestines? Despite common feelings that bacteria are disgusting and dirty, some bacteria are strong, valiant species that are effective at protecting your body from harmful substances you ingest. Certain bacteria are particularly excellent knights; these bacteria are called lactic acid bacteria, a type of probiotic. There are many types of probiotics worthy of being knights. Lactic acid bacteria such as Lactobacilli and Bifidobacteria are worthy knights, as are some yeast species like *Saccharcomyces boulardii*.

Probiotics offer a great number of health benefits. Probiotics guard the intestinal lining protecting the gates to your body from harmful substances. Probiotics also strengthen your gates by promoting a healthy intestinal lining; they are involved in a variety of reactions in the body that stimulate the immune system helping you stay healthy. Also, probiotics limit the growth of pathogenic microbes in the intestinal tract, keeping you healthy. In many studies, lactic acid bacteria has flexed its muscle and shown how it helps protect the host against pathogens. By doing so, lactic acid bacteria acts as a shield, protecting you against the negative effects of unfriendly microbes such as *E. coli*, Salmonella and *Candida albicans*. In other words, probiotics are like knights that protect the intestines from ransacking invaders.

FORTIFIED BY FOOD

These friendly microbes are consumed orally in breast milk, vegetables, dairy products and other foods. In the days before antibacterial and food processing, humans ate lots of foods that contained microbes. Some of these microbes were unhealthy; modern processing techniques that limit our exposure to these harmful microbes are beneficial to our health. However, some of the bacteria and yeasts we used to eat in our foods were good for us. Sauerkraut, kimchi, kefir, kvass, miso, beer, wine and tamari are all foods that are made with the help of bacteria and yeast. The most common source in your diet of probiotics is likely yogurt and cheese. New probiotic-rich foods have been emerging on the market since 2000, including probiotic chocolate bars, cereals, milks and more. To date, the best way to get high dosages of probiotics into your gastrointestinal tract is through probiotic supplementation. Probiotic supplementation supplies billions of live active cells to the intestines, which is far more than can be added to most food products. We take a more in-depth look into probiotic foods and supplements in Chapter 18.

How Do Probiotics Work?

The exact mechanisms of action by which probiotics elicit their beneficial effects are not fully understood. Researchers are working to better understand the specifics of these proposed mechanisms by which probiotics appear to affect the health of humans. Here are some of the known mechanisms by which probiotics can elicit their beneficial effects in the human gastrointestinal tract.

Probiotics Compete for Receptor Sites
This mechanism can be thought of as drivers fighting for parking spots in a small lot. Once in the intestinal tract, probiotics strive to reach the receptor sites along the epithelial cells that line the intestines. Epithelial cells, which line the intestinal tract, mouth and vagina, are host to millions of receptor sites for various microbes. Some probiotics are very effective at attaching to receptor sites. In other words, some probiotics are like aggressive drivers that are good at finding parking spaces. One of the main selection criteria used by scientists when looking for probiotics to use in foods and supplements is their ability to attach to receptor sites. Good probiotics can find open parking spots in a lot, thus preventing bad microbes from finding space. Probiotics literally "crowd out" the bad microbes. Of note, some probiotics can

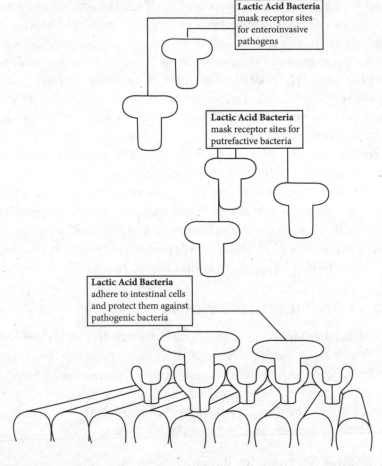

Figure 3-1 shows labels:

Lactic Acid Bacteria mask receptor sites for enteroinvasive pathogens

Lactic Acid Bacteria mask receptor sites for putrefactive bacteria

Lactic Acid Bacteria adhere to intestinal cells and protect them against pathogenic bacteria

Figure 3-1: Mechanisms by which Lactic Acid Bacteria (Probiotics) Inhibit Bad Microbes from Attaching to Your Cells.

affect bad microbes' ability to adhere to a receptor, in the same way you can make it hard for a car to park in the space beside yours if you park on an angle or very close to the line.

Probiotics Mask Receptor Sites

When probiotics bind to a receptor site on an epithelial cell, they elicit a number of effects in the cell. One of the proposed effects is that probiotics communicate with the cell, causing the cell and its neighboring cells to alter their lining. The lining of the intestinal tract is covered in mucus, similar to your nose. This mucus lining of the intestinal tract helps protect the intestinal wall from invading pathogens. When probiotics cause a positive change to the lining, bad microbes are less able to attach.

The cells that line the intestinal tract appear to be able to cross-talk, allowing for a communal exchange. Cells have junctions between them called "tight junctions." Through these junctions scientists think that cells communicate to each other, which enables them to react as a group. When a probiotic tells one cell to change to prevent bad microbes from attaching, the cell can then tell all of its neighbors to do the same. The result is a large protective change that protects the body from infection and creates immunity. When pathogens cannot adhere to the intestinal receptors, they cannot colonize and cause disease.

Researchers Lu and Walker have suggested that probiotics strengthen tight junctions between intestinal cells, which ultimately improves immunity.

Probiotics Affect the Immune System

Probiotics positively affect the immune system in a number of ways, but we do not yet completely understand how they do what they do. There are two parts to your immune system: innate and acquired. Probiotics enhance both of these. They also increase the production of compounds (certain cytokines) that promote good inflammation. In the intestinal tract, probiotics cause the intestinal lining to be less permeable, which means that harmful microbes and toxins that are not supposed to enter into your bloodstream cannot do so. Let's take a closer look at this area of research.

The gastrointestinal tract is the main entry for pathogens into your body. Just think about the number of bacteria and chemicals you ingest each day. As such, your gastrointestinal tract is lined with its own set of immune cells to help prevent these harmful substances from gaining entry to your body. These immune cells are called the gut-associated lymphoid tissue (GALT). The GALT is the largest mass of immune tissue (**lymphoid tissue**) in the human body and as such is an important element of the body's immune system. You may be familiar with other lymphoid tissues such as the tonsils and spleen. The tonsils are also located in an area where you are commonly exposed to harmful substances (the throat). Your immune tissues are in locations where you need them most, such as your intestinal tract, throat, nose and lungs. They may not physically touch each other, but they stay in close communication with each other by producing protein-messengers, such as **antibodies** and **cytokines**. Antibodies are proteins that help the body tag or identify unwanted items, called **antigens**. When a bad microbe or substance (antiges) interacts with the intestinal lining, the immune cells produce antibodies (e.g., Immunoglobulin A[IgA]).

The ability of the immune tissues to communicate allows an immune response initiated in the GALT to affect other immune tissues, such as the lungs. In other words, a response to an antigen (e.g., peanuts) in the digestive tract could cause an effect in the lungs such as shortness of breath and tightening of the throat, as seen in **anaphylactic shock**. It is not surprising that researchers are discovering that probiotic supplementation is useful in a wide variety of immune-based ailments including allergies, asthma, eczema and irritable bowel disease.

The gut microflora is an important part of the intestine's defense barrier. This is known because where there is no microflora more antigens are able to get across the intestinal lining and gain access to the body. In other words, when there are no probiotics present, the defense barrier is weak. To simplify further, without knights out front to protect your castle, it is more susceptible to invading pillagers.

Probiotics appear to reduce the severity of some allergic reactions such as anaphylaxis and asthma. It is not fully understood how this happens, but scientists think that probiotics help balance good and bad messengers of the immune system by keeping the system in check. The result is healthy immune reactions and a healthier you. A careful balance of inflammation is required in the intestinal tract. Too much of an immune reaction can result in inflammation and damage to the intestines reducing their ability to digest and absorb nutrients, and can also lead to the development of diseases such as irritable bowel disease. Too little immune reaction allows pathogens to grow in the intestines, causing infectious diarrhea, which can develop into a chronic illness such as allergies or an autoimmune disease without the anti-inflammatory effect of specific strains of probiotics.

All in all, it appears that probiotics:

- reduce allergic reactions
- improve overall immunity
- promote proper immune reactions against pathogens.

Probiotics are great helpers to the immune system in the intestines and appear to support proper immune reactions throughout the body.

Probiotics Consume Available Nutrients

The intestines are the ideal environment for lactic acid bacteria to grow. There are lots of nutrients available in the digestive tract that support the needs of lactic acid bacteria to grow. By consuming a large portion of the available nutrients suitable for microbes, lactic acid bacteria restrains the growth of bad microbes. With little to eat, pathogens find it hard to grow and colonize in the intestines.

Probiotics Create an Acidic Environment

Lactobacilli and Bifidobacterium are bacteria families that excrete lactic acid and acetic acid into their environment. This excretion of acid is part of their regular daily functions. In the gastrointestinal tract, this causes the pH to lower. Many bad microbes do not like a low pH. As such, lactic acid bacteria are capable of inhibiting the growth and colonization of bad microbes in the gastrointestinal tract.

Probiotics Produce Beneficial Enzymes

Probiotics make a variety of enzymes that offer health benefits to you. These enzymes include lactase, which breaks down lactose, a sugar in milk that many people cannot digest. Some probiotics produce enzymes that are harmful to bad microbes. The enzyme activity of probiotics has been found to help fight infectious disease, lactose intolerance, immune system deficiencies, and urogenital and vaginal diseases.

Probiotics Produce Antimicrobial Effects

Some probiotics have antimicrobial effects. Many of the probiotic strains of bacteria are able to produce substances that kill bacteria, called **bacteriocins** such as lactocidin, reuterin or acidophilin. These bacteriocins have antimicrobial activities that reduce the growth of disease-causing microbes. To date, only some strains are known to to produce antimicrobial substances. *L. reuteri*, *L. plantarum* and *L. casei* are examples of clinically studied probiotic species that have antimicrobial effects and can produce bacteriocins. Each antimicrobial substance appears to target certain bad microbes. As more antimicrobial substances are discovered, scientists will be able to recommend specific probiotic species for the nasty microbes humans encounter, including *E. coli* and *C. difficile*. Perhaps then, if you eat *E. coli*–contaminated spinach, you could use a probiotic to help fight the *E. coli* in your system.

Probiotics Support Gut Barrier

Lactobacilli and Bifidobacteria produce fats that encourage the growth of cells that line the intestinal tract. These fats are called **short chain fatty acids**. These fats also have nutritional effects on the intestinal cells, keeping them well nourished and healthy. Probiotics help with the proper maintance of the gut barrier function by helping keep intestinal cells healthy.

Probiotics Encourage Healthy Microflora

Probiotics may also work synergistically to create an environment that promotes probiotic growth, not growth of bad microbes. Some probiotics excrete substances that enhance the growth of fellow probiotics. *Lactobacillus reuteri* excretes AGGH, a protein that appears to encourage growth of good bacteria in the small intestine. This is a fascinating area of research. In clinical trials, the use of combinations of probiotic species has been found to offer greater health benefits than any one of the probiotic species alone. As such, it is likely that probiotics work synergistically in the intestines to promote the growth and colonization of fellow friendly microbes.

BYE, BYE BAD BUGS

It's like the Wild West in your intestines. Probiotics are the sheriff and they're saying to the bad microbes, "There ain't enough room in this intest-town for the two of us." Which bug will reign supreme in your gut? Say goodbye to bad bugs because one of the most unique attributes of probiotics is their selective ability to promote the growth of friendly bacteria in the human digestive tract, while inhibiting the growth of pathogenic ones. There are many mechanisms by which probiotics inhibit the growth of bad bacteria in the human digestive tract:

1. Competitive nutrient consumption
2. Epithelial cell receptor interactions
3. Excretion of antimicrobial substances
4. Interaction with the immune system.

These mechanisms and other actions of probiotics were discussed in detail earlier in this chapter. So let's move on and investigate how probiotics work against specific bad microbes.

Candida

Everyone's body is host to Candida (*Candida albicans*). Candida is a type of yeast. Candida is normally kept under control by good health and probiotics. However, Candida overgrowth can occur when the system is challenged or altered. The use of antibiotics can reduce the ability of probiotics to keep Candida at bay. Also, the overconsumption of yeast-feeding foods such as simple carbohydrates, sugars, peanuts, alcohol and milk products can encourage Candida growth.

Candida overgrowth can elicit a number of symptoms, the worst of which is the burning, itching symptoms associated with a vaginal candida overgrowth, also known as a yeast infection or vulvovaginal candidiasis (VVC). The development of VVC is associated with a lower number of Lactobacilli in the vagina, particularly those which produce hydrogen peroxide. Hydrogen peroxide is a chemical that kills bacteria. The presence of hydrogen peroxide in the vagina would kill bad microbes like Candida.

To date, there is some argument as to the ultimate effect of hydrogen peroxide producing Lactobacilli in the control of Candida in the vagina. In vitro (test tube) studies have shown that Lactobacilli can inhibit the growth of *Candida albicans* and its adherence on the vaginal lining. Clinical trials (human studies) support the effectiveness of Lactobacilli, especially *Lactobacillus acidophilus*, *Lactobacillus rhamnosus* and *Lactobacillus fermentum*, administered either orally or intravaginally. These probiotics colonize in the vagina and prevent the growth of *Candida albicans*.

Lactobacillus crispatus and *Lactobacillus jensenii* are capable of displacing the well-known vaginal pathogens *Candida albicans* and *Gardnerella vaginalis*. All of these probiotic species are effective in inhibiting *Candida albicans* growth, reducing its ability to attach to vaginal cells. There is more research required in this area and it is likely that there are more probiotic species that can effectively inhibit *Candida albicans* infections in the vagina.

Candida overgrowth in the vagina, also known as a yeast infection, is perhaps the most common Candida problem. Candida also lives in the gastrointestinal system, where it can cause havoc. In the mouth it can cause thrush in infants, and in the intestines it can cause a gamut of problems. Some experts believe that an overgrowth of Candida in the intestines is common and causes what is referred to as the "yeast syndrome." Physical symptoms include fatigue, headache, mood swings, sinus congestion, depression, poor memory and concentration, and cravings for sweets. The 1980s book *The Yeast Connection* made the public aware of yeast growth control and catapulted Candida into a mainstream health concern. It is thought that the following factors contribute to Candida overgrowth: use of oral contraceptives, steroids, antacids, ulcer medications, antibiotics, high-sugar diets, pregnancy, smoking, food allergies or intolerances and diabetes. Luckily, Lactobacillus probiotics are capable of keeping *Candida albicans* under control in all areas of the body.

The mouth is host to a large number of microbes including *Candida albicans*. As Candida overgrowth is a particular problem in the elderly, a double-blind, placebo-controlled study investigated the effects of eating a probiotic cheese daily for four months. The study included 276 elderly people and found the probiotic was successful in reducing the risk of high yeast counts by 75%. In other words, probiotic bacteria are effective in controlling Candida in the mouth, a problem of particular concern for the elderly.

The exact mechanism by which probiotics inhibit Candida growth is not fully understood to date. Some suggest the ability of probiotics to produce hydrogen peroxide plays a role; however, in vivo studies suggest that probiotics might prevent Candida growth through multiple mechanisms.

E. coli

Escherichia coli O157:H7 (*E. coli*) is a leading cause of foodborne illness. People can become infected with *E. coli* in a variety of ways. Though most cases have been associated with eating undercooked, contaminated ground beef, people have also become ill from eating contaminated bean sprouts or fresh leafy vegetables such as lettuce and spinach. Person-to-person contact in families and childcare centers is also a known mode of transmission. In addition, infection can occur after drinking raw milk and after swimming in or drinking sewage-contaminated water.

Based on a 1999 estimate, 73,000 cases of infection and 61 deaths occur in the United States each year. Infection with *E. coli* often leads to bloody diarrhea and occasionally to kidney failure. Once digested, *E. coli* attaches to the host epithelial cells and causes detrimental changes to them. Probiotics can positively change the cells that line the intestines so that bad bacteria such as *E. coli* cannot live there.

Many species of probiotics have traits that might help rid an intestinal tract of *E. coli*; however, clinical trials have found that *L. acidophilus* is the superior probiotic for an *E. coli*–infected intestine. It can effectively inhibit the growth and ability of *E. coli* to attach to the intestines. Thus, this pathogen cannot thrive in the intestinal tract. *L. rhamnosus* is also respected as an effective probiotic for infected human intestinal tracts.

H. pylori

Helicobacter pylori (*H. pylori*) is the most common bacterial infection in developing countries and often results in chronic gastritis (inflammation of the stomach), peptic ulcers and gastric cancer. *H. pylori* is a bad bacterium that can inhabit the cells that line the stomach. Many who are infected do not show any symptoms of disease. The *Helicobacter spp.* are the only known microbes that can thrive in the highly acidic environment of the stomach. Treatment of an *H. pylori* infection typically involves the use of antibiotics, commonly two, and omeprazole, a pharmaceutical used to reduce acid production in the stomach. By completely eliminating *H. pylori*, the harm of the infection, typically peptic ulcers, can heal. Therefore, getting rid of this bacteria infection is a way to regain health.

Probiotics are able to prevent infection by *H. pylori*. Research in animal models has shown probiotics prevent infection from this nasty bacterium. Researchers have found that pretreating animals with probiotics reduces the ability of *H. pylori* to infect them. The probiotics were also able to reduce the inflammation caused by an *H. pylori* infection. Less inflammation means less pain and damage to the stomach. Based on this and other research, probiotics are thought to be an effective defense against infection from *H. pylori*.

The ability of probiotics to prevent against an *H. pylori* infection has yet to be confirmed in humans; however, probiotics are effective in treating people who are already infected. A half-dozen clinical trials investigating the ability of probiotics to treat people with *H. pylori* infections have showed a positive result.

It is a difficult task to **eradicate** *H. pylori* in the stomach. For a probiotic to be a good treatment for *H. pylori* infections it would have to be tolerant to the low pH of the stomach and have the ability to attach to the unique lining of the stomach. *L. acidophilus*, *L. gasseri* and *L. rhamnosus* show potential as effective probiotics to fight *H. pylori* infections and invasions. Another successful probiotic is *L. reuteri*. In Italy, researchers investigated the ability of *L. reuteri* to eradicate *H. pylori* in a double-blind, placebo-controlled study of 30 infected people. A dosage of only 800,000 (8×10^5) CFUs was administered twice daily, along with omeprazole to the infected subjects. The study found that *L. reuteri* was able to stop *H. pylori* infections by reducing the ability of *H. pylori* to attach to the stomach lining. As such, there appear to be a number of probiotic species that may be useful in the prevention of *H. pylori* infections and potentially in the eradication of an infection.

Rotavirus

Rotavirus is the pathogen responsible for infantile diarrhea, winter diarrhea, the stomach flu, acute nonbacterial infectious gastroenteritis and more. Seven major groups of Rotaviruses have been identified, three of which infect humans. Rotaviruses cause vomiting and diarrhea. The virus infects the villi, which are small, finger-like projections on the small intestine. Rotavirus causes a change in the villi structure that results in diarrhea. It is the most common cause of severe diarrhea in children, killing about 600,000 children every year in developing countries. The incubation period ranges from one to three days. Symptoms often start with vomiting followed by four to eight days of diarrhea. Recovery is usually complete; however, severe diarrhea without fluid and electrolyte replacement may result in death.

The probiotic *Lactobacillus rhamnosus* GG is effective in promoting a rapid recovery of watery diarrhea in children with a Rotavirus infection. The exact way this probiotic helps children get better has not been discovered; however, preliminary research suggests that *L. rhamnosus* GG may increase cell production in the small intestine which acts to wash out cells that are infected with the virus. Removing the virus from the body shortens the duration of diarrhea.

Diarrhea in children can be life threatening: there is a research study that is worth noting. Children (aged one month to three years) with acute-onset diarrhea were enrolled in a double-blind, placebo-controlled study. The children were randomly divided into two groups, one to receive placebo or *Lactobacillus rhamnosus* GG. Probiotic dosages were at least ten billion (10^{10}) CFU. Children receiving the probiotics had a significant reduction in the duration of their diarrhea (56 hours versus 77 hours in the placebo group) and hospital stays were significantly shorter in the probiotic group. This study and others support the use of *Lactobacillus rhamnosus* GG in children with acute diarrhea as a safe way to shorten the duration of their diarrhea and reduce the time they have to be in the hospital.

L. reuteri is another probiotic known to help with diarrhea. Two double-blind, placebo-controlled research trials looked at the effects of *L. reuteri* in children with acute infectious diarrhea. Daily dosages of one hundred billion (10^{11}) CFU of *L. reuteri* was well tolerated and effectively prevented diarrhea in the young children. The probiotic significantly reduced diarrhea symptoms to only one and a half days. In another study, newborns were supplemented with *L. reuteri*. The newborns had no evidence of adverse effects and experienced a significant reduction in the incidence of watery diarrhea. In these trials, many children had confirmed Rotavirus infections causing the diarrhea. A large number of clinical trials support the use of *L. reuteri* to reduce the severity and duration of diarrhea.

Salmonella
Salmonella is one of the major causes of foodborne illness worldwide. Every year, approximately 40,000 cases of Salmonella

infections (poisoning) are reported in the United States. Because many milder cases are not diagnosed or reported, the actual number of infections may be thirty or more times greater. Young children, the elderly and those with weak immune systems are most likely to have severe Salmonella infections. It is estimated that approximately 600 persons die each year with acute Salmonella infections. There are many different kinds of Salmonella bacteria with Salmonella serotype *typhimurium* and Salmonella serotype *enteritidis* being the most common in the United States.

Salmonella is a type of bacteria that lives in the intestinal tracts of humans and other animals. As such, Salmonella is usually transmitted to humans by eating foods contaminated with feces. Many raw foods of animal origin are frequently contaminated, but fortunately, cooking kills Salmonella. Improper hand washing by food handlers is another source of contamination. Of note, Salmonella can also exist in animal feces and thus pet owners, including reptile owners, should be careful to wash their hands after handling pets and/or their excrement.

Animal researchers are working with probiotics to see if they can help reduce the presence of Salmonella in the feces of farmed animals to reduce the likelihood of human food contamination. At the University College in Ireland, researchers divided pigs into two groups, one of which received regular milk, while the other received milk containing five probiotic strains. Following six days of treatment, the pigs were exposed orally to Salmonella bacteria and their health was then monitored for 23 days. The pigs that had received the probiotic treatment had fewer incidences, less severe, and shorter durations of diarrhea, as well as significantly lower numbers of Salmonella in their fecal samples. Thus, administration of probiotic bacteria appears to improve the outcome of Salmonella infection in pigs and may help reduce the likelihood of human infection from contaminated food.

In Canada, researchers at the University of Guelph investigated the ability of probiotics to prevent Salmonella infection in broiler chickens. The researchers found that pre-administration with probiotics (*Lacobacillus acidophilus, Bifidobacterium bifidum and Streptococcus faecalis*) enhanced the chicken's immune response. The probiotic supplement chickens had superior health. Prebiotics were also investigated in this trial, and they were found only to be of added health benefit when probiotics were given simultaneously. It appears that probiotics can prevent Salmonella's growth in many animals commonly farmed for human consumption.

These animal studies have shown a number of probiotic species are capable of preventing Salmonella from growing. Two other probiotics, *S. cerevisiae* and *L. reuteri* can inhibit the growth of Salmonella, according to laboratory-style research trials. As a result, it appears that the use of probiotics in farmed animals may help reduce their illness and the possibility of food-contaminated cases of Salmonella among the general human population.

To date, there are no clinical trials on probiotic use in the prevention and treatment of Salmonella infections in humans. However, animal studies offer promise that probiotics may play a role in the prevention and treatment of Salmonella infections in humans.

There are many bad microbes that probiotics are known to fight. Appendix 3-1 lists a number of human disease conditions, along with the corresponding microbe that causes each condition, and the probiotic shown in scientific studies to destroy it.

BIFIDOBACTERIA AND BAD BACTERIAL INFECTIONS

Most of the probiotic species mentioned above are of the Lactobacillus family. This is because many bad microbes like to inhabit the small intestine where lactobacilli like to live. However, the large intestine is also a location in which bad microbes try to live. As such, Bifidobacteria also play an important role in preventing infections. Bifidobacteria has been shown in a number of research trials to protect the body from intestinal infections that can cause illnesses such as diarrhea.

We know that infants with high numbers of Bifidobacteria can resist certain infections by bad microbes. The elderly are not as able to withstand infection. Could this be due to the decrease in the number of Bifidobacteria in our colon that occurs as we age? As the number of Bifidobacteria decreases, the number of *Clostridium perfringen*, a bad microbe, increases. *C. perfringen* strains produce a variety of toxins and volatile amines. Toxins and volatile amines can cause damage to the colon causing inflammation, constipation and potentially cancer.

Luckily, supplementation with Bifidobacteria has been shown in clinical studies to substantially decrease the number of *clostridium* in the elderly and to promote colon health.

Bifidobacteria are great at reducing the growth of bad microbes in the colon. *B. longum* is one probiotic known to help fight Salmonella *typhimurium* infections. There are many bad microbes that can be controlled by Bifidobacteria. Appendix 3-2 lists bad microbes known to be inhibited by species of Bifidobacteria.

SUMMARY

Once probiotics reach their receptor sites, they serve as a protective shield along the intestinal mucosa. They are able to inhibit the ability of bad microbes to attach and grow in the intestines. Some probiotics can produce antimicrobial or synergistic substances that kill bad microbes and promote the growth of friendly microbes respectively. Probiotics also consume nutrients, thus reducing those available for bad microbes and thereby limiting their growth. These many ways that probiotics reduce the ability of bad microbes to live and grow in your intestines promote a healthy intestinal lining.

Bye, bye bad bugs. Probiotics have a unique ability to inhibit pathogenic microbe adhesion, invasion and colonization in the human body. Pathogens such as *E. coli*, Salmonella and Rotavirus cause serious illness at high frequency among the human population. Candida, a natural inhabitant of the human body, can cause havoc if allowed to grow uncontrolled. Lactobacilli and Bifidobacteria have illustrated the ability to inhibit the invasion and growth of all of these nasty microbes.

As well, probiotics support the immune system and thus enhance the body's ability to fight these pathogens. Their effect on the immune system goes even farther. Probiotics have positive effects on the immune system, which keeps it functioning properly.

Probiotics can be used as prevention against infection or overgrowth of bad microbes to support overall health, and research indicates they can also be used to effectively treat pathogenic microbe infection.

chapter
4

Not Created Equal: Probiotic Species and Strains

A MICROSCOPIC VIEW OF THIS CHAPTER

- A probiotic is identified by genus, species and strain.
- Probiotic strains can be found in a variety of microbial genuses.
- Lactobacilli love the small intestine; Bifidobacteria love the colon.
- The origin of a probiotic can tell you some of what it does.
- Transient probiotics have health benefits, but do not colonize in the body.
- Different ages require different probiotics.
- Each species of probiotic has its own set of health benefits.
- Multispecies are most effective.
- Different strains of probiotics have different characterisitics.

■ ■ ■ ■ ■ ■ ■

SORTING AND CLASSIFYING MICROBES AND PROBIOTICS

Considering there are over a quadrillion (10^{14}) microbial species in your intestines, it's appropriate that we identify the different species and what they do. When discussing types of microbes, we use **taxonomical** classifications to help identify them. First, the **genus**, or family name, tells us that the microbe shares a common set of characteristics. For example, Bifidobacteria is the name of the genus and this genus has the characteristic of being able to produce lactic acid, and it has a Y-shape. Second, the **species** tells us more specifics about the microbe. For example, describing a bacterium as *Lactobacillus acidophilus* tells you it is of the genus Lactobacilli and the species *acidophilus*. All *acidophilus* species share a subset of characteristics that makes them different from other species of Lactobacilli. Third, we can describe a specific bacterium even further by describing the **strain**, which is commonly noted by a series of letters and/or numbers. For example, *E. coli* 0157:H7 is a specific strain of bacteria. Each strain of bacteria has its own characteristics that are unique to it alone.

genus > species > strain

Probiotics are not a genus, species or strain. The term *probiotic* is used to describe a group of microbes that offer benefits to you, the host. Microbes that behave as probiotics can be found in different genuses: Bifidobacterium, Lactobacillus, Streptococci, Enterococcus, Saccharomyces and Lactococci. Of note, not every species in these genera act as probiotics. In other words, not every Enterococcus species is a probiotic. In Appendix 4-1, you will find a list of common probiotic species found in commercial products that are commonly the subject of scientific research. Let's take a closer look at the probiotics found in these four genera of bacteria.

Probiotics can be found in the Bifidobacteria genus. Bifidobacteria are normal inhabitants of the human colon and are also found in many animal species. In fact, it only takes a few days after birth for the colon to be colonized with Bifidobacteria, particularly breast-fed infants. Bifidobacteria were first isolated in the feces of breast-fed infants. This family of bacteria appears to colonize and remain at stable population levels in humans until advanced age (elderly) when its population numbers seem to decline. Bifidobacteria can produce lactic and acetic acids, and as such are also classified as lactic acid bacteria. Bifidobacteria are also found in the human vagina. Probiotic species in the Bidifobacteria family include *B. lactis*, *B. bifidum* and *B. longum*.

Lactobacilli are another family of bacteria that normally live in the human intestine, mouth and vagina. Capable of producing lactic acid, Lactobacilli are classified as lactic acid bacteria. This ability to produce lactic acid has been put to use in the production of yogurt as *Lactobacilli acidophilus* is a primary bacteria in yogurt products. Probiotic species in the Lactobacilli family found in the human body include *L. reuteri*, *L. casei* and *L. rhamnosus*.

Streptococci are also found in dairy products. *Streptococci thermophilus* is commonly used to make yogurt. Some Streptococci species are probiotics. *Streptococcus salivarus* **subspecies**, *thermophilus*, is a probiotic found in the human mouth, throat and nasopharynx and is thought to offer healthy benefits to humans.

Enterococcus is another family of bacteria that occupies both animal and human intestinal tracts. Enterococcus is a lactic acid–producing bacteria. Two species are commonly found in the intestines of humans: *E. faecalis* (90–95%) and *E. faecium* (5–10%). These two species of Enterococcus have probiotic effects in humans.

Saccharomyces belongs to the yeast family or genus. Saccharomyces is from the Latin meaning "sugar fungi." Many members of this genus are considered very important in food production. One example is *Saccharomyces cerevisiae*, which is used in making wine, bread and beer. *Saccharomyces cerevisiae* is more commonly known as baker's yeast. I will leave it up to you to decide which name you'll use from now on; however, referring to this vital baking ingredient as *S. cervisiae* may make you sound smart at parties. *Saccharomyces boulardii* is the principle probiotic yeast noted in the media and in commercial products. *S. boulardii* is normally beneficial to the body and has been used to treat diarrhea associated with antibiotic use and *C. difficile*.

Lactococci is another genus that includes some probiotic species. Lactococci are classified as lactic acid bacteria as they can introduce lactic acid to their environment. *Lactococcus lactis* (formerly known as *Streptococcus lactis*) is found in dairy products and is commonly responsible for the souring of milk.

You can find a wide variety of these probiotics in foods and supplements around the world. Appendix 4-1 lists probiotic species commonly found in commercial products.

Probiotic Origins

Commercially used probiotic strains have been isolated from vegetable, animal or human origins. The origins of each strain will vary. The origin can help tell you a bit more about the product. A probiotic from animals and vegetables is more likely to be **transient.** Transient probiotics travel through the intestinal tract, eliciting some health benefits, but they do not attach and colonize in the body. Human strains are typically great colonizers. The more likely a probiotic is to colonize, the greater the resulting duration and potency of its health benefit. *NOTE:* Some products on the market use soil-based probiotics, which are not usually the same strains as those used in clinical trials and are not of human origin; thus, they may not offer you the same health benefits.

THE TWO MOST POPULAR GENUSES

The two most popular probiotic genuses are Lactobacilli and Bifidobacteria. These are the most common genuses in probiotic foods and supplements around the world. Let's take a closer look at these two probiotic families.

There are twice as many Bifidobacteria in the human intestinal tract than Lactobacilli. Bifidobacteria reside predominantly in the lower intestine where they elicit most of their health benefits. As the colon or large intestine is the final stage of food digestion it is full of Bifidobacteria's favorite food: incompletely digested carbohydrates, e.g., inulin, fructoolgiosaccharides, which are also called prebiotics. Bifidobacteria are capable of readily fermenting these carbohydrates. In the large intestine, Bifidobacteria can inhibit the growth of bad microbes via multiple mechanisms including the ability to lower the pH of the environment by excreting lactic acid and acetic acid. Bifidobacteria are also important for the production of thiamine (B1), riboflavine (B2), pyridoxine (B6), folic acid, cyanocobalamine (B12) and nicotinic acid. The B vitamins are required for energy production. If you are feeling sluggish, it is often due to a deficiency in B vitamins. They also play a role in your mood. Bifidobacteria are vital for the proper health of the lower intestine and your feelings of overall wellness.

Both Lactobacilli and Bifidobacteria may be lactic acid–producing bacteria; however, they differ in shape, and they prefer to live in different locations in the human intestinal tract. Lactobacilli are rod-shaped and Bifidobacteria are Y-shaped. Bifidobacteria like to live in the colon, while Lactobacilli like to live in the small intestine.

Both families of bacteria are capable of inhibiting bad microbes in their favored environment; however, their mechanisms can vary slightly. Lactobacilli produce lactic acid but do not produce acetic acid like their Bifidobacterium cousins. Lactobacilli bacteria are also different in that some species can excrete chemicals that act as antimicrobials. Through a number of mechanisms, Lactobacilli can promote the healthy colonization of probiotic species in the intestinal tract. Lactobacilli are also effective at promoting the health of the cells that line the intestines and keep the immune system in line and working correctly. It is the latter of these health benefits of the Lactobacilli genus that are unique to this genus.

Known Species of Lactobacilli and Bifidobacteria
Lactobacillus (Family: Lactobacilli)
Lactobacillus acidophilus
Lactobacillus amylovorus
Lactobacillus brevis
Lactobacillus bulgaricus
Lactobacillus casei
Lactobacillus casei sp. *rhamnosus*
Lactobacillus crispatus
Lactobacillus delbrueckii
Lactobacillus fermentum
Lactobacillus gallinarum
Lactobacillus jensenii
Lactobacillus johnsonii
Lactobacillus plantarum
Lactobacillus reuteri
Lactobacillus rhamnosus
Lactobacillus salivarius
Lactobacillus sporogenes
Lactobacillus vaginalis

Continued

Bifidobacteria (Family: Actinomycetaceae)
Bifidobacterium adolescentis
Bifidobacterium animalis
Bifidobacterium bifidum
Bifidobacterium breve
Bifidobacterium infantis
Bifidobacterium lactis
Bifidobacterium longum
Bifidobacterium regularis (trademarked
name for *B. animalis* DN173 010)

WHICH PROBIOTIC SPECIES ARE BEST FOR YOU?

In the young, evolving science of probiotics, there are always more questions than answers. Knowing exactly which species are right for you will likely be a question we cannot accurately answer for many years to come. However, there are a few generalizations we can make that can help you find the right probiotic species for you.

GENERA VARY

As these two genera are the most popular on the market, understanding their differences can help determine which one may offer you the best health benefits. Remember where these probiotics like to live. Lactobacilli live in the small intestine and are helpful in treating diarrhea, some inflammation-based conditions, promoting a healthy immune system and improving digestion. Vaginal problems can be targeted with Lactobacilli as this genus likes to live in the vagina and is known to promote health in this area of the body.

You can choose a probiotic based on its preferred location to live in the intestinal tract.

Bifidobacteria live in the colon and thus are very helpful in improving health of the colon, including relieving constipation. We know that as we age the levels of Bifidobacteria in our colon tend to drop resulting in health problems. The result of low Bifidobacteria colonies in the colon of the elderly is an increase in constipation episodes, presence of bad microbes and the production of toxins by these microbes which can be **carcinogenic**.

As such, ensuring your diet contains the Bifidobacteria genus of bacteria may be beneficial to health in the elderly.

Appendix 4-2 illustrates the presence of Bifidobacteria species in infants and adults. *It is wise to choose a probiotic based on your age requirements.* Notice the change in the makeup of the species present with age. In the elderly, a change in cell receptors or environmental factors may be the cause of the decreased presence of Bifidobacteria in their colon. Children's probiotic supplements focus on the species known to inhabit a healthy infant's intestines, such as *L. rhamnosus* and *B. infantis*. Supplementing with probiotic species based on age is another way to choose a probiotic.

EACH SPECIES OF PROBIOTIC HAS ITS OWN HEALTH BENEFITS

Different species of probiotics offer different health benefits. For example, despite being from the same genus, *L. acidophilus* and *L. reuteri* do not have the same health benefits in the human body. Yes, both have antimicrobial effects, which reduce the presence of bad microbes in the intestines; however, *L. acidophilus* has additional health benefits including the ability to produce vitamin K and lactase. As such, *L. acidophilus* has a different set of health benefits than *L. reuteri*. Does this mean that *L. acidophilus* is superior to *L. reuteri*? That is difficult to measure as each species has a different set of health benefits; it is like comparing apples to oranges. *L. reuteri* can inhibit bad microbes in the intestines, as *L. acidophilus* can; however, *L. reuteri* can excrete reuterin, a potent antimicrobial shown in clinical studies to effectively treat cases of Rotavirus diarrhea and *H. pylori* infections. Thus, both species of Lactobacilli are very beneficial. Each has its own set of health benefits—each set is equally important to overall human health. As you can see, it is not easy to decide which probiotic is better than another.

There probably is no one ultimate probiotic species for health; there is no magic bullet. Each probiotic offers a different set of health benefits. As well, you can get a synergistic effect by having many different probiotic species in your intestinal tract.

In research trials, combinations of probiotics have been found to be more useful than a single species alone. For example, *L. rhamnosus* and *L. reuteri* are better at alleviating **acute** diarrhea than a single probiotic species. Probiotic species work better together than alone. If probiotics could sing to us, perhaps they would sing, "So, happy together."

STRAINS ARE DIFFERENT

Have you ever wondered why sometimes a species of probiotic appears twice on a product label? When this happens, there is a series of letters and numbers after the species name. This indicates that there are different strains of that probiotic species present in the product. Each species of bacteria, e.g., *L. acidophilus*, has strains, e.g., *L. acidophilus* HA-122 and *L. acidophilus* M92. In other words, when we refer to a species of probiotics, it is actually a group of bacteria strains. Each strain can exhibit different characteristics or health benefits. For example, *Lactobacillus acidophilus* HA-122 is a particular strain of this species that is particularly resistant to acid. As such, this strain is used in some probiotic supplements that are taken orally and its acid resistance allows it to successfully pass through stomach acid on the way to its preferred destination—the small intestine.

When looking at the ingredient label of a probiotic food or supplements, you can identify the strain by the series of letters and numbers that follow the species name. Particular strains may offer better health benefits than others. Clinical research papers will specify which strain was used.

If you want to use probiotics to target a particular illness, be sure to get the exact strain indicated in the research studies. A similar strain may not produce the same health effects.

As the science of probiotics is still in its infancy it can be difficult to find a clinically researched probiotic strain on the supermarket shelves for every disease condition. Only some conditions have been sufficiently studied to know which strains or even species are most effective.

Researchers have investigated whether particular probiotic species are effective against a specific disease conditions. For example, *L. plantarum* has been clinically studied for its effects against irritable bowel syndrome. *L. salivarius* has been studied to see if it inhibits the growth of *Helicobacter pylori*, a bacterium found in the stomach and associated with some ulcer formation. In both cases, researchers found these specific probiotic species to be effective against the targeted disease condition. There are many examples of studies where probiotic species have been used to target a disease condition; however, not every species has been tested against every disease. The result is some areas of diseases are well studied and others less. In Part II, we will dive into the research in this area. We'll investigate what scientists have found when they have researched the effect probiotics may have on a wide variety of disease conditions. A short summary of this information is captured in Appendix 6-2.

Most of us are looking for a particular strain to make our shopping experience a little easier. What shall we do then? Remember that a healthy, balanced intestinal microflora can offer you many healthy benefits. Experts are recommending the use of a variety of probiotic species (and strains) to promote optimal health.

MULTI-SPECIES PROBIOTICS ARE BEST

A multi-species probiotic is highly recommended based on current knowledge about probiotics and their health effects. Why is this? Combinations of probiotic species have been found to have a synergistic effect. In other words, species of probiotics work together to give a greater health benefit than a single species can alone. Let's look at an example. A combination of *L. casei, L. plantarum, L. acidophilus, L. bulgaricus, B. longum, B. breve, B. infantis, S. thermophilus,* known as VSL#3, has been used in a number of clinical trials along with single probiotics. In most cases, the combination of a number of probiotics offered an increased health benefit (synergisitic effect). Multi-species supplements are better for your health.

Most multi-species probiotic products on the market contain Lactobacilli and

Consuming a combination of probiotic species can offer a wide range of health benefits.

Bifidobacteria species, but new species and genera are being assessed for future use. The future will likely unveil many more probiotic species that may offer even greater health benefits. Watch for new technology in the future that increases the viability of probiotic species to enable more convenient ways for ingestion including more shelf-stable techniques to be used in both supplements and foods.

SUMMARY

A probiotic species is identified by its genus, species and strain. The genus is a family name like Bifidobacteria. A species such as *acidophilus* identifies that the probiotic has a set of characterisitics. Each strain of probiotic has its own unique characteristics. Which probiotic species is right for you? You can choose a probiotic based on its preferred location to inhabit in the body or by your age requirements. For example, Lactobacilli love to live in the small intestine and Bifidobacteria love to live in the colon. In some disease conditions, researchers know which specific species offers health benefits. However, there is much research left to be completed. If choosing a probiotic strain based on its effects in clinical research, be sure to purchase the exact strain—different strains have different effects. Experts agree that having a healthy mixture of a variety of probiotic species in the intestinal tract can provide the best health benefits. In other words, multi-species probiotics may be the right choice for you. In Chapter 18, we'll discuss in more detail how to find the right probiotic food or supplement for you. In Part II, we'll discover what health benefits probiotics can offer and which offer the best health benefits for which disease conditions.

chapter
5

Prebiotics: Food for Probiotics

A MICROSCOPIC VIEW OF THIS CHAPTER

- Prebiotics are carbohydrates, food for probiotics.
- Prebiotics support growth and activity of healthy intestinal microflora.
- Bifidobacteria are simulated by prebiotics, called the bifodogenic effect.
- Prebiotics lower blood cholesterol and triglyceride levels.
- Prebiotics may have positive effects on calcium absorption and cancer prevention.

■ ■ ■ ■ ■ ■ ■

Despite how similar in spelling prebiotics is to probiotics, the two are very different. Only probiotics are living organisms. Prebiotics are actually carbohydrates. Prebiotics are carbohydrates that the body cannot digest, but probiotics can! Since the body cannot digest prebiotics, they are left unaltered as they travel through the intestinal tract and reach the colon ready to be used by the probiotics living there, particularly Bifidobacteria. Prebiotics are the preferred food source for probiotics. Prebiotics are nondigestible oligosaccharides (a short-chain sugar molecule) that help promote the growth and activity of probiotics.

What is an example of a prebiotic? Inulin, beta-glucan, pectin and resistant starch are all carbodhydrates that act as prebiotics in the human intestinal tract. Inulin is found in onions, chichory root and dandelions; oligosaccharides are found in artichokes, leeks and asparagus; beta-glucan is found in seaweed, oats and barley; pectin is found in apples and apricots; and resistant starch is found in raw bananas, potatoes and beans. Research has shown that eating prebiotics can improve the growth of lactic bacteria in your intestines, especially Bifidobacteria. Prebiotics also help to inhibit the growth of a variety of undersirable microorganisms.

Prebiotics are non-digestible food ingredients that may beneficially affect the host. Prebiotics selectively stimulate the growth and activity of one or a limited number of good bacteria in the colon and thus improve the host's health.

Prebiotics are naturally present in our daily diets; however, the Western diet does not include sufficient prebiotics to properly support our probiotic flora. Our diet is about two to three times too low in prebiotics. It has been estimated that North Americans eat about 1 to 4 grams of prebiotics (e.g., inulin and other oligosaccharides) daily, while Europeans consume 3 to 10 grams per day. Humans should consume at least 4 grams of prebiotics each day. We eat too many processed foods, sugary treats and meats.

WHAT FOODS CONTAIN PREBIOTICS?

Flax, barley, oats and other whole grains are great sources of prebiotics. Greens, such as spinach, kale and dandelion leafs, are also a good source of prebiotics. Prebiotics can be found in lentils, including chickpeas and kidney beans. Even delicious favorites like berries and bananas are natural sources of prebiotics.

Since prebiotics are not digested by the body, they have a reduced caloric value. They do not lead to a rise in your blood glucose level or stimulate the secretion of insulin. What they do offer is fiber. Prebiotics are dietary fiber. As such, they have many positive effects on your intestines. Fiber helps to increase stool frequency, particularly in people suffering from constipation. Prebiotics also decrease fecal pH. This drop in pH helps prevent the production of harmful (putrefactive) substances by bad microbes in the colon. By this mechanism, prebiotics may have a cancer preventative effect. These harmful chemicals can lead to damage of colon cell DNA, which can, in turn, lead to cancer.

Do you need another reason to include prebiotics in your diet? Researchers have found that the consumption of prebiotics decreases the level of bad fats in your blood. In a research trial, the blood levels of triglycerides and cholesterol decreased with prebiotic use in people with high cholesterol levels.

Do you need fiber for your bones? Yes. Prebiotics have been shown in animal studies to have positive effects on calcium absorption. Prebiotics (inulin and oligofructose) may contribute to the prevention of osteoporosis. Eat more grains, greens, beans and berries as these prebiotic foods may offer a whole array of healthy benefits.

You might not find raw, green bananas appealing for dinner, but your microflora do. Raw, green bananas are a great source of resistant starch. Ripe bananas do not have the same amount of resistant starch. Resistant starch is an area of prebiotics that is gaining interest within the research world. Preliminary results suggest that resistant starch may increase the ability of probiotics to survive through the stomach. This means a larger number of probiotics can make it safely to their preferred site (small or large intestine) when prebiotics are in your diet. Resistant starch has a bulking capacity that may modify stomach pH and dilute the bile acid level in the small intestine. The ability of resistant starch to help probiotics survive the way down to the small and large intestine, added to its ability to beneficially stimulate the growth of microbes in your colon, has this prebiotic high on the up-and-coming supplement list.

> **What is the Difference Between Dietary Fiber and Prebiotics?**
> Both are non-digestible fiber. Prebiotics selectively promote the growth of colonic microbes. Prebiotics are dietary fiber; however, dietary fiber does not promote the growth of probiotics.

POPULAR PREBIOTICS

The most popular prebiotics are short chain fructooligosaccharides, more simply referred to as scFOS or FOS. Inulin is a type of FOS. The only difference between FOS and inulin is the number of chains in their chemical structure. Inulin and FOS are commercially available in foods and supplements. Inulin and FOS are synthesized from the sugar of beets and extracted from chicory root, respectively. By the way, chicory root is the root of the Belgian endive plant.

FOS is thought to be one of the best prebiotics. This is because other prebiotics (inulin and other oligosaccharides such as oligofructose) have to be converted by the human body before they can be used by the probiotics. FOS does not need to be converted. Prebiotics requiring metabolism are considered to be less effective than FOS. FOS is ready to offer its healthy benefits the instant it is consumed.

How do prebiotics work? In essence, the fundamental concept is the same for prebiotics as for probiotics. Prebiotics improve your health by beneficially affecting the intestinal microflora. In other words, prebiotics improve the makeup of the intestinal flora so that you stay healthy. Prebiotics support good microbes and inhibit the bad. The use of prebiotics alone can actually change the makeup and activity of the intestinal microflora.

The probiotic family, Bifidobacteria, are the common target for prebiotics. Why is this? Oligosaccharides are the preferred food source of Bifidobacteria. As such, prebiotics are sometimes referred to as having a **bifidogenic** factor, as they support the growth and colonization of Bifidobacteria. Please note that prebiotics may sometimes be referred to as "fermentable substrates." This is because Bifidobacteria break down prebiotics with a process called fermentation to create energy.

Bifidogenic Effect

A product that stimulates, or claims to stimulate, Bifidobacteria is said to have a bifidogenic effect on the intestinal flora. Inulin, FOS and other prebiotics are known to have a bifidogenic effect in humans.

Synbiotics

Researchers are looking at the effect of combining probiotics and prebiotics in what is called a **synbiotic**. Synbiotics, both probiotics and prebiotics together, are thought to produce more beneficial health effects than either on their own. This may be because prebiotics promote the growth of existing probiotics in the colon and improve the survival and growth of newly added probiotic strains. Prebiotics are the perfect, supportive partner for probiotics.

The European Union is sponsoring a project called SYNCAN that is looking into possible cancer-protective effects of synbiotics. The project was sparked by animal models that have shown that synbiotics dramatically reduce the development of cancer. The research says that synbiotics are more powerful than their prebiotic or probiotic components alone. Results from the SYNCAN project are promising. A human trial from the project found that a combination of inulin, *Lactobacillus rhamnosus* and *Bifidobacterium lactis* reduced the risk of colon cancer. As more results from SYNCAN are released, it will likely spark an increase in symbiotic products on the market.

Combining probiotics with prebiotics has already been welcomed by the food industry. In Europe, there are many dairy drinks and yogurt manufacturers combining both in products such as Aktifit (Emmi, Switzerland), Probioplus (Migros, Switzerland) and Fyos (Nutricia, Belgium), to name a few. Watch for more research in this area, particularly studies that identify which probiotic strains and prebiotic combinations are most effective. This is an exciting new area for prebiotics.

As prebiotics are so easily manufactured and are a part of a well-known food group (fiber), the general public is very accepting of prebiotic food products. Keep your eyes open for new food products that have added FOS, inulin or other prebiotics. Check out supermarket shelves for breads, cereals, fruit bars and perhaps soon even ice creams containing prebiotics.

SUMMARY

Prebiotics are carbohydrates that the human body cannot digest. When prebiotics are consumed in foods such as berries, beans, greens and grains, these carbohydrates reach the colon unaltered. There they are fermented by resident probiotics, Bifidobacteria. Prebiotics support the growth and health of probiotics. A prebiotic is capable of enhancing probiotic health and inhibiting the growth of bad microbes. Ultimately, prebiotics improve your health. Prebiotics lower blood cholesterol and triglyceride levels as well as having positive effects on calcium absorption and cancer prevention. The effect of probiotics can be enhanced when taken with prebiotics, a combination described as a symbiotic.

PART 2

Probiotics to the Rescue

chapter
6

From Diarrhea to Constipation: Probiotics and the Toilet

A MICROSCOPIC VIEW OF THIS CHAPTER

- Diarrhea can be acute or chronic.
- Acute diarrhea is caused by an infection of bad microbes.
- Probiotics prevent the ability of bad microbes to infect the intestinal tract.
- Certain probiotics reduce the severity and duration of diarrhea.
- By improving immunity in the intestinal tract, probiotics can prevent diarrhea.
- Antibiotic use destroys probiotics and increases the risk of diarrhea.
- Probiotics can be used at the same time as antibiotics.

■ ■ ■ ■ ■ ■ ■

No matter whether you call it a lavatory, the ladies' room or the porcelain throne, no one enjoys being uncomfortable on the toilet. Diarrhea and constipation are among the top complaints about the digestive tract. Do you suffer from these toilet woes?

Diarrhea can be the most dangerous health problem of these two intestinal issues. One hundred million people are affected with acute diarrhea each year in the United States. Perhaps this explains why there are so many jokes about the toilet in Western society. Unfortunately, diarrhea is no joking matter—particularly, when you realize that of the one hundred million affected with diarrhea each year about three thousand people die from it. Diarrhea is not just a major health problem in North America; it is a global issue. A large proportion of the world's population, even in developed countries, is affected by foodborne diarrhea. Sadly, a majority of the deaths globally occur among children in the developing world.

The average adult has a bout of acute diarrhea about four times a year.

People of all ages can get diarrhea. In the United States, each child will have had seven to 15 episodes of diarrhea by age five, and the average adult is afflicted with acute diarrhea four times a year.

WHAT IS DIARRHEA?

Diarrhea is loose, watery stools. Typically, a person with diarrhea will pass stool more than three times a day. Acute (short-term) diarrhea is very common and usually goes away without any medical help in one to two days. Diarrhea may be accompanied by cramping, abdominal pain, bloating, nausea and/or an urgent need to use the bathroom. Depending on the cause, a person may have a fever or bloody stools.

Can Diarrhea Kill?

Diarrhea caused by a bad microbe (bacteria, virus or parasite) can result in death. The bad microbe can sufficiently damage the intestines to cause severe diarrhea, dehydration and drastically reduce nutrient absorption to a point where the body cannot get enough vital nutrients and water to survive. This is not common; however, if diarrhea is left untreated or if the pathogenic species is unresponsive to treatment, death can occur.

Generally, there are four types of diarrhea: acute diarrhea, traveler's diarrhea, antibiotic-associated diarrhea and chronic diarrhea.

Acute Diarrhea

Acute diarrhea is a term used to describe a short period of loose stools. The cause can vary from foreign microbe or parasite ingestion, consumption of spoiled foods, use of antibiotics or infection by a virus.

Traveler's Diarrhea

Traveler's diarrhea is a common term used to describe acute diarrhea in a person who has consumed water or food contaminated with bacteria, viruses or parasites when visiting a foreign location. This is not common in Canada, the United States, Australia, New Zealand or most European countries.

Antibiotic-Associated Diarrhea

Antibiotic-associated diarrhea is a type of acute diarrhea. Antibiotics are very effective at eliminating bacteria from the body. They are helpful if there is an overgrowth of bad (pathogenic) bacteria that causes illness such as Strep throat or a urinary tract infection. However, antibiotics are not selective about which bacteria they clean out of the body. Probiotics are also destroyed with antibiotic use. After antibiotic use, the body is more susceptible to infection by bad microbes because there is a low level of probiotics which normally defend the body from invasion. Diarrhea caused by bad microbes after antibiotic use is called antibiotic-associated diarrhea. This can be a serious problem in the elderly and children.

Chronic Diarrhea

Chronic diarrhea may be a sign of a more serious problem. Chronic diarrhea is usually related to a functional problem in the intestines such as irritable bowel syndrome or inflammatory bowel disease. Chronic diarrhea poses the risk of dehydration, the very risk that puts the elderly and children at risk of death. Dehydration is a condition in which the body lacks enough fluid to function properly. To avoid serious health problems, dehydration should be treated quickly. All individuals suffering from diarrhea should focus on rehydrating the body.

WHAT CAUSES DIARRHEA?

There are many things that can cause diarrhea. Appendix 6-1 provides a list of potential causes of diarrhea. Acute diarrhea is usually due to a bacteria, virus or parasite infection. When a bacteria, virus or parasite is able to flourish in the intestines, it causes damage to the intestinal cells. How do they cause damage? Bad microbes produce toxic chemicals, which they release into the intestines. These toxins cause damage to the cells that line the intestines. The result is swelling or inflammation of the intestinal walls and diarrhea. These toxins damage the microvilli of the small intestines. The microvilli are finger-like projections that absorb nutrients. The longer the villi are, the more surface area there is for absorption of nutrients from you gut into your bloodstream. In other words, long villi are key to a healthy body. Damage to intestinal cells (including those which make up the villi) by bacteria, viruses or parasites reduces the body's ability to absorb nutrients and water. The result is faulty water absorption, which causes diarrhea and dehydration.

Diarrhea is responsible for several million deaths around the globe each year. It is a major world health problem. It is thought that predisposition to infections (e.g., diarrhea) is associated with immaturity and improper functioning of the intestinal barrier. In other words, the lining of the intestine is unable to keep bad microbes away from the intestinal cells. Probiotics help promote a healthy, strong intestinal barrier. As such, the use of probiotics can help to prevent and treat diarrhea. Bifidobacteria and other lactic acid bacteria have been shown in research trials around the globe to protect the body against the devastating effects of diarrhea.

ACUTE DIARRHEA IN CHILDREN

Probiotics can help stop diarrhea in children. This is not news. We've read about it in the newspaper for over a decade. The most well-known effect of consuming probiotics is their ability to reduce the severity and duration of diarrhea in children. Early studies were done in Asia with heartwarming results. Resolving acute diarrhea in children is of great importance in third-world countries where infants commonly drink bacteria-, virus- and parasite-contaminated water, which leads to diarrhea and even death.

Acute infantile diarrhea is often the result of an infection by the Rotavirus. Children with a Rotavirus infection have fever, nausea and vomiting, which are often followed by abdominal cramps and frequent, watery diarrhea. Children who are infected may also have a cough and runny nose; however, as with all viruses, all or few of these symptoms may appear.

Rotavirus is particularly common in the winter. In North America and other

Rotavirus most often infects infants and children, aged three months to two years.

countries with a temperate climate, Rotavirus has a winter seasonal pattern, with annual epidemics occurring from November to April.

Since Rotavirus is stable in the environment, it can easily be transferred from person to person. It is typically transferred by fecal–oral transmission. Rotavirus moves from one human to another by ingestion of contaminated water or food and contact with contaminated surfaces. All it takes is one person forgetting to wash his or her hands after going to the washroom and then proceeding to prepare a salad for dinner.

Many research studies have investigated which probiotic species can prevent and treat acute diarrhea in children. *Bifidobacterium bifidum, Bifidobacterium breve, Bifidobacterium lactis, Lactobacillus rhamnosus* and *Lactobacillus reuteri* are known to have positive health benefits in children who are infected with Rotavirus. Appendix 6-2 summarizes the clinical evidence on the ability of probiotic strains to fight diarrhea in children and infants. Let's look at some of this research in more detail.

As diarrhea can be so devastating, an obvious population group to target in studies is children hospitalized with diarrhea. Here are the particulars on two such research studies that involved children suffering from diarrhea.

Studies of Probiotics for Treatment and Prevention of Diarrhea in Children

In a clinical trial, 69 children who were hospitalized for acute diarrhea in Denmark were randomized to receive either a 10 million CFU mixture of *Lactobacillus rhamnosus* and *Lactobacillus reuteri* or **placebo**, twice daily for five days. Both of these strains have been shown to have probiotic characteristics in in vitro (test tube studies) and in healthy adults. The combination of *L. rhamnosus* and *L. reuteri* resulted in a 48% reduction in the hospitalization rate and effectively reduced diarrhea in the children. We know that probiotics can help fight diarrhea in healthy adults and in infected children.

This second study offers a measure of how much probiotics help alleviate diarrhea in children. In two hospitals, a prospective, randomized, placebo-controlled trial was conducted. The trial involved children between the age of six and 36 months with Rotavirus-associated diarrhea. The children were randomized into three groups and received either placebo or 10 billion or 10 million CFUs of *L. reuteri* once a day for up to five days. The duration of watery diarrhea was greatly reduced in those receiving the *L. reuteri* supplementation. The large dose (10 billion CFU) had a more profound effect on shortening the duration of watery diarrhea than the smaller dosage. In fact, only 48% of the children receiving the higher dosage of probiotics had watery diarrhea by the second day of treatment, versus 70% of those receiving the small dosage and 80% of those in the placebo group. This study tells us two things:

1. *L. reuteri* appears to shorten the duration and severity of Rotavirus-associated diarrhea in children as young as six months of age.
2. The effectiveness of probiotics depends on the dosage.

   Please note that all of the research to date suggests that probiotics have the best effects on your health when you consume dosages of at least 10 million to 10 billion (10^7 to 10^9) CFUs.

Probiotics do not just help children fight off a Rotavirus infection; they may also offer a preventative effect. *L. casei* was shown in a multicenter research trial in France in 2000 to effectively reduce acute diarrhea incidence in children. In another trial, both *Bifidobacterium bifidum* and *Streptococcus thermophilus* were given in a milk formula to infants and was found to reduce the number of times the children got sick with a Rotavirus infection. Bifidobacterium breve has also shown the ability to prevent infections of Rotavirus in children. As we can see, there are many studies showing that probiotics, when taken regularly, can help prevent children from getting sick with Rotavirus infections.

Can Probiotics Help Children in a Daycare Setting?

In 2002, a group of Danish researchers decided to look into the ability of probiotics to help children with acute diarrhea attending daycare centers. The children were supplemented with 10 million (10^7) CFUs of *L. rhamnosus* and *L. reuteri* twice daily for five days. The children taking the probiotic recovered twice as fast as those receiving the placebo. Thus, the researchers concluded that a combination of *L. rhamnosus* and *L. reuteri* is effective at shortening the duration of acute diarrhea in daycare children. It would appear, based on all of these studies, that probiotics can help prevent children from getting diarrhea, even in high-risk locations like daycare centers and help them feel better, faster when they do become ill with diarrhea.

Is One Probiotic Species Better Than Another?

Few studies have directly focused on whether one species is better than another in treating acute diarrhea in children. One study compared a Lactobacilli strain to a Bifidobacteria strain. *L. reuteri* was compared to *B. lactis* and to a placebo in a prevention study in childcare centers in Israel. *L. reuteri* was effective at reducing the severity of the children's diarrhea. It was more effective than *B. lactis*. As Lactobacilli species love to live in the small intestine, the location of the diarrhea infection, it is likely that these species would be most effective in treating diarrhea.

Is there one species of Lactobacilli that is better at preventing diarrhea than others? *L. rhamnosus* strain GG (also called *L. casei*) was compared with *L. rhamnosus Lactophilus*. *Lactobacillus rhamnosus* GG was more effective in reducing the quantity of watery stools after the first day of treatment, while *L. rhamnosus Lactophilus* was not. These observations suggest that different species of Lactobacilli have different abilities to treat diarrhea. Unfortunately, we do not yet know which probiotic is best at treating diarrhea. Further studies are needed.

The Role of Yogurt

What about using yogurt as a treatment for acute diarrhea in children? The literature is split: some studies suggest yogurt is helpful and some do not. However, there tends to be a trend in the research that yogurt can shorten the duration of diarrhea in children.

Yogurt may offer some benefit in acute diarrhea in children.

Lactobacilli are used as starter organisms to make yogurt; thus it is not surprising to think of yogurt as a treatment for diarrhea. On the other hand, children can have undetected food intolerances and allergies to dairy products. Giving yogurt to these children to treat diarrhea may make the problem worse. Using yogurt to help alleviate acute diarrhea in children should be reserved for those known to be toleratant to dairy products.

There are many more clinical studies that have investigated the effect of probiotics on children with acute diarrhea. In fact, it could almost be a book in itself. Appendix 6-2 offers a summary of these studies. We can conclude that both Lactobacilli and Bifidobacteria can help prevent and even treat acute diarrhea in children, and a number of species appear to be effective.

ANTIBIOTIC-ASSOCIATED DIARRHEA

In our bacteria-phobic world, packed with antibacterial dish and bathroom soaps, antibiotics are considered a miracle drug to many. However, the overuse of antibiotics and antibiotic products has resulted in some negatives, including the development of antibiotic-resistant bacteria and a rise in antibiotic-associated ailments. Antibiotic-resistant bacteria, or superbugs, are discussed in more detail in Chapter 16. One the most severe side effects of antiobiotic use is antibiotic-associated diarrhea.

Antibiotics are commonly used in developed countries to treat illness. Antiobiotics are drugs that kill bacteria. Some people are using antibiotics for illnesses that are not caused by bacteria, such as the common cold, which is caused by viruses. A national survey of Canadians done by Ipsos-Reid discovered that 30% of consumers believe that most colds and flus can be treated successfully with antibiotics. This is incorrect. Most colds and flus are caused by viruses and as such would not be aided by antibiotics. This misconception causes an overuse of antibiotics, which in turn leads to an increased number of cases of antibiotic-associated diarrhea.

This prevalent consumer belief that antibiotics can treat the common cold may explain the high use of antibiotics in developed countries. Also, physicians are over-prescribing antibiotics. When asked, 53% of Canadian consumers said they had been prescribed an antibiotic in the previous three years. That is a lot of antibiotic use.

Antibiotics are very effective at killing bacteria in the body; however, you will recall that antibiotics do not kill just the bacteria that is making you sick. Antibiotics kill both the bad and the good bacteria. While antibiotics destroy the bad bacteria that is making you sick, they also kill the probiotics that are vital to your health and your immunity.

Antibiotics do not just kill most of the probiotics in your body; they also affect their ability to colonize. This means that probiotics cannot grow when you are taking antibiotics. The result is a compromised microflora in your intestines. Without probiotics, bad microbes can invade you and cause illness. Most commonly, the bad microbes cause diarrhea, hence the term antibiotic-associated diarrhea.

About 39% of patients who receive antibiotics will develop diarrhea.

Antibiotic-associated diarrhea is a common problem. The incidence of antibiotic-associated diarrhea in hospitals has been found to range from 3% to 29%. Antibiotic-associated diarrhea has been associated with an increased number of days of hospitalization and higher medical costs. Probiotics are an attractive option for preventing antibiotic-associated diarrhea as they are becoming increasingly available, are low in cost and have a lack of side effects. As probiotics don't have the problems associated with antibiotics, they are becoming a popular way for people to prevent bacterial infections, thus reducing the need for antibiotic use.

The gastrointestinal tract is the major portal of entry of pathogens.

Probiotic Therapy and Antibiotics

Probiotic therapy involves using probiotics to balance the microflora and thus helps the intestinal barrier prevent infection from bad microbes. This type of therapy is particularly important when antibiotics are used because the natural healthy balance of microflora has been drastically altered. In other words, when you take antibiotics it kills off your natural defenses in your intestines, and this is a problem. The intestines face the most attacks from bad microbes; your intestines are the major entry point into your body for pathogens. Research has uncovered a unique interaction between the intestines and probiotics. Probiotics help the intestinal lining fight off attacks from bad microbes.

What Types of Bad Microbes Do We Ingest?

We have already seen that Rotavirus is an example of a bad microbe that can have grave consequences: it causes diarrhea. However, any bad microbe can attach to an intestinal cell and colonize there, releasing toxins and causing damage that leads to diarrhea. It is particularly easy for a bad microbe to attach to your intestinal cells if antibiotics have washed away the probiotics which normally prevent infection of bad microbes.

Probiotics successfully prevent antibiotic-associated diarrhea.

Antibiotic-associated diarrhea can be the result of an overgrowth of *Clostridium difficile*, a bad microbe that lives in your intestines. Normally, probiotics keep this nasty microbe under control and it is not allowed to grow and cause you to feel ill. The changes that antibiotics cause

---

A Deadly Bacteria

Clostridium difficile (*C. difficile*) is a type of bacteria that can be found in human feces. When antibiotics kill your good intestinal bacteria, *C. difficile* is allowed to grow. When it grows, *C. difficile* produces toxins that damage the intestines and may cause diarrhea.

C. difficile disease is usually mild but sometimes can be severe. In severe cases, surgery may be needed, and in extreme cases *C. difficile* may cause death. Symptoms include watery diarrhea, fever and abdominal pain or tenderness. It is the most common cause of infectious diarrhea in hospitals or long-term care homes. Who gets *C. difficile*? It usually occurs after the use of antibiotics. Old age, presence of other serious illnesses and poor overall health may increase the risk of severe disease. Diagnosis of *C. difficile* disease can be done with a simple stool test and it is commonly treated with antibiotics. However, probiotics would be beneficial in this probiotic poor intestinal situation.

C. difficile is spread by fecal–oral contaimination. Bacteria in the stool can contaminate surfaces such as toilets, handles, bedpans or commode chairs. Hand washing is vital to reducing the spread of this potentially deadly disease. Read more about this illness and how probiotics can help in Chapter 16.

to the intestinal environment offers *Clostridium difficile* a chance to flourish. Since antibiotics can reduce the ability of probiotics to colonize, antibiotic use can commonly lead to growth of bad microbes such as Clostridium. This is a major problem in elderly people and can lead to serious diarrhea and at times death.

Probiotics for Prevention of Antibiotic-Associated Diarrhea

It is wonderful that probiotics can help alleviate antibiotic-associated diarrhea; however, can probiotics prevent antibiotic-associated diarrhea? Yes, they can. In 2002, a group of scientists reviewed all of the research available on the ability of probiotics to prevent antibiotic-associated diarrhea. This type of review is called a meta-analysis. The review consisted of nine randomized, double-blind, placebo-controlled trials—the gold standard of trials. The researchers concluded that probiotics can be used successfully to prevent antibiotic-associated diarrhea; in particular the probiotics *L. acidophilus*, *Enterococcus faecium*, *L. bulgaricus* and *S. boulardii* have the best potential in this situation. Two of the trials included children.

Bifidobacterium longum has also been shown to reduce the number of times and length of antibiotic-associated diarrhea. An interesting strain, *Bifidobacterium bifidum*, is actually able to neutralize the toxins that bad microbes produce. This means that the toxins cannot damage your intestinal cells and that translates into no more diarrhea.

Which specific strains are best for antibiotic-associated diarrhea has not yet been conclusively determined by the scientific community. However, species of both the Bifidobacteria and Lactobacilli genus have shown promise as supportive tools in reducing the loss of immune strength in the intestinal tract during health challenges, including antibiotic use. As such, probiotics are a possible way of preventing antibiotic-associated diarrhea. The relative lack of side effects makes probiotics even more attractive in the use of antibiotic-associated diarrhea.

Certain probiotic strains have been found to reduce the incidence of *Clostridium difficile* infection when taken concurrently with antibiotics; however, these strains have not yet been shown to directly treat a *Clostridium difficile* infection. *Clostridium difficile* produces toxins that cause a series of symptoms in the host. This particularly devastating condition, which is causing havoc in cities across North

America, including Montreal, will be discussed in more detail in Chapter 16.

| *Probiotics can be taken with antibiotics.* Can you take a probiotic at the same time as an antibiotic? In all nine of the trials reviewed in the meta-analysis above, probiotics were given at the same time as antibiotics. In fact, a number of the studies noted that probiotics can offer you health benefits even when they are taken at the same time as antibiotics. *S. boulardii* is a well-known probiotic that can reduce the severity and duration of diarrhea caused by antibiotic use. This is because *S. boulardii* can quickly cause changes to cells in your intestine that helps them fight off any invading bad microbes. Clinicians who are experts on probiotics are suggesting that a probiotic be taken at the same time as an antibiotic. They do not mean in the same mouthful, as the antibiotic would kill the probiotic before it has a chance to help you. Clinicians suggest taking your probiotic and antibiotic about four hours apart to reduce their interaction. Four hours is plenty of time for a probiotic to have time to attach to your intestinal cells. If you happen to take them closer together, you would not lose all of the benefits of the probiotics. One mouthful of antibiotics cannot kill all of the probiotics in your body; thus, if you keep replacing your probiotics between dosages of antibiotics, you will always have some probiotics present to help you fight off bad microbes that can cause diarrhea.

In conclusion, antibiotics kill the probiotics in your body, reducing your ability to fight off bad microbes that can cause diarrhea. Research has found that probiotics, including *Saccharomyces boulardii*, Bifidobacteria and Lactobacilli can destroy bad microbes, help the body defend itself (boost immunity) and thus prevent and treat diarrhea associated with antibiotic use. Probiotics can be taken at the same time as antibiotics.

PROBIOTICS FOR TREATING INFECTIOUS DIARRHEA

Probiotics are effective at fighting infectious diarrhea. This is done through a number of mechanisms:

- Promoting the production of mucous by intestinal cells acting like fly-tape and making it hard for bad microbes to attach to these cells
- Competing with bad microbes for binding sites on intestinal cells and nutrients needed to help them grow
- Producing acidic substances that lower the pH of the intestines, something not liked by bad microbes
- Increasing intestinal movement, which means bad microbes get carried out with the feces and cannot sit around and grow in your intestines.

Probiotics also turn on genes that control innate immunity, which further contributes to the elimination of pathogens. Perhaps one of the most fascinating things that some probiotic strains can do is produce bacteriocins (antimicrobials)—substances that kill bad microbes in your intestines. They function like home-made antibiotics that do not kill probiotics. For example, *Lactobacillus* GG can produce an antimicrobial substance that prevents the growth of the following bad microbes: *Escherichia coli*, Salmonella, *Clostridium difficile*, *Bacteroides fragilis* and Streptococci. For more information on the mechanisms by which probiotics affect the immune system and help your intestines become a barrier that prevents bad microbes from infecting you, see Chapter 3.

Some probiotic strains have antibiotic-like actions but do not kill probiotics.

PROBIOTICS FOR TREATMENT AND PREVENTION OF TRAVELER'S DIARRHEA

No one likes to travel with a roll of toilet paper in their purse. However, it is true: travelers commonly suffer from acute diarrhea. Medical professionals would say, "Ingestion of foreign bacteria and viruses can cause acute diarrhea." What they mean is that if you eat a bad microbe on your travels that your body has not seen before, you're less able to fight it off and can end up with diarrhea. No one visits the buffet at their favorite resort with a microscope hoping to identify any microbes that might be living on the fruit salad. Let's face it—avoiding foreign microbes when traveling is virtually impossible. Hand washing can eliminate a certain amount of exposure; however, it may not be enough.

Acute diarrhea can be a particular problem for travelers visiting areas in which there are low hygiene standards. If repeated hand washing and careful food choices do not prevent exposure to bad microbes, luckily there are probiotics that can help you. Probiotics can attack these invaders before they attach, colonize and cause diarrhea. The good news is that probiotics can help you prevent getting traveler's diarrhea.

Research studies have found that probiotics can prevent bad microbes from causing traveler's diarrhea. The ability of a probiotic to prevent traveler's diarrhea is dependent on many factors including the strain of the probiotic, the number of strains/species used, the destination of the traveler and the way in which the bad microbe causes diarrhea. *L. rhamnosus* GG and *S. boulardii* have been shown in three double-blind, randomized control trials to offer a preventative effect against acute diarrhea commonly picked up when traveling. These two species of probiotics are good items to include on your next packing list.

Researchers are not convinced that there is enough evidence to support a medical recommendation to use probiotics to prevent traveler's diarrhea. They still suggest that the best way to prevent traveler's diarrhea is to practice proper hygiene. Yes, this is true; however, why not double-up on your protection? Research suggests that probiotics offer some protection to travelers, particularly those in high-risk areas. More studies may help us make a more concrete recommendation to travelers to use probiotics as a means to prevent diarrhea. I always include probiotics in my vacation bathroom kit.

SUMMARY

Diarrhea is a major health problem that affects people of all ages and health conditions. Diarrhea is a particular problem in children and the elderly as it reduces their ability to absorb nutrients and can cause them to become dehydrated. There are two types of diarrhea: chronic and acute. Chronic diarrhea is usually due to a problem with the intestines' ability to function, such as irritable bowel disease. Acute diarrhea is caused by an infection. In the intestines' bad microbes can produce toxins that damage the cells of the microvilli (finger-like projections on the lining of the small intestine that are responsible for most of the nutrient absorption by the body). The damage caused by these toxins leads to diarrhea. Probiotics are effective in the management and potentially in the prevention of diarrhea. Probiotics help the intestinal cells prevent bad microbes from attaching and causing an infection. There have been three meta-analyses (reviews of all of the research available) looking at the ability of probiotics to help fight diarrhea. The studies used in the review were all of high quality—double-blind and placebo-controlled. There is a convincing amount of evidence that supports ths use of probiotics to prevent and treat cases of acute diarrhea in children, antibiotic-associated diarrhea and traveler's diarrhea. For the prevention and treatment of diarrhea, probiotics are a safe, effective option.

chapter
7
Probiotics for Infants

A MICROSCOPIC VIEW OF THIS CHAPTER

- A mother's microflora influences the child's.
- A different microflora is found in children than adults.
- Breast-feeding introduces important probiotics and pre-biotics to an infant.
- Infant formulas should include probiotics and prebiotics to promote health.
- Probiotics can treat and prevent childhood diarrhea.
- Probiotics reduce the number of sick days taken by day-care children.
- Probiotics play an important role in a child's immunity.
- Colic can be helped by probiotics.
- Clinical trials show probiotics are safe in children as young as four months of age.

■ ■ ■ ■ ■ ■ ■

Birth is arguably the most miraculous event on earth from at least a biological perspective. A baby develops in the mother's uterus from just two cells. When a baby is born, it passes through the birth canal and is introduced to the outside environment. Because the uterus is sterile, a newborn child does not have the 400 species of microbes that typically live in a healthy human. A newborn infant is first introduced to microbes in the birth canal. Very quickly, infants develop a diverse microflora. How does this happen? Which species are most important to an infant's health? Do probiotics play a role in infant immunity as they do in adult immunity? Let's discover more about the important relationship between infants and probiotics.

MOM, PROBIOTICS—AND BABY MAKES THREE

Initially, a newborn's microflora is strongly dependent on the mother's microflora, the way the baby is born (natural or C-section) and the environment the baby is born in. A mother's microflora can influence a baby's health in the womb in a number of ways. A mother's probiotic flora helps with the production of vitamins essential for infant development. Probiotics inhibit bad microbes in the vagina from causing infections that can cause early labor. Probiotics also promote proper immune reactions in the mother, preventing the mother from having negative immune reactions that can harm the baby.

The most important benefit of the mother's probiotics (maternal microflora) for the growing fetus is their ability to fight bad microbes. The maternal microflora prevents the growth of bad microbes in the vaginal tract; however, sometimes this is not enough and infections occur. It is estimated that vaginal infections cause up to 30% of preterm labour. Bacterial vaginosis is the medical term used to describe a negative change in the types of microbes in the vagina. Bacterial vaginosis usually develops when there is a drop in the number of Lactobacilli in the vagina. Lactobacilli are normally present in high quantities in the vagina where they help to keep bad microbes at bay. *Gardnerella, Escherichia coli* and other bad microbes naturally live in very low numbers in the vagina. When the number of Lactobacilli drops, these bad microbes are allowed to grow. What increases the risk of developing bacterial vaginosis? Vaginal douching, stress and antibiotic use increase the risk of developing bacterial vaginosis.

Treatment of bacterial vaginosis with antibiotics decreases the incidence of preterm labor, according to preliminary studies. Probiotics may be a safe alternative to antibiotics for treatment and they may even prevent bacterial vaginosis. Evidence suggests that Lactobacillus plays an important role in maintaining the health of the urinary and reproductive tract. In 2006, a research study was initiated at Mount Sinai Hospital in Toronto to investigate the effects of Lactobacilli in preterm labor. The results of this study (not released at time of publication) may offer some insight into the use of probiotics to prevent preterm labor caused by bacterial vaginosis in at-risk mothers.

Bacterial Vaginosis

Symptoms of bacterial vaginosis include pain, discharge and itching. Bacterial vaginosis is commonly mistaken for yeast infection and is commonly self-treated with over-the-counter antifungals. This misdiagnosis and mistreatment of bacterial vaginosis can have bad consequences. The use of antifungals to treat bacterial vaginosis is not very successful; cure rates are as low as 60%. The major problem is that bad microbes can overgrow in the vagina without proper treatment. Probiotics may offer assistance as they can reduce populations of bad microbes in the urogenital tracts without adverse reactions.

YOUR BABY'S MICROFLORA

The microflora of a newborn develops rapidly after birth. At birth, the microbes that live in the cervix of the mother are introduced to the infant. In fact, a 1979 study found that the stomach contents of a five-minute-old baby reflected the microbes found in the cervix of the mother. Non-vaginal births can reduce the introduction of probiotics found in the vagina to newborns and, unfortunately, there is no known way to get the same microflora into babies that are born this way.

Bacteria starts to appear in the feces of newborns within 24 hours after birth. Bad microbes such as *Escherichia coli* and Enterococci are frequently found in early stool samples of newborns and commonly are identical to strains found in their mother.

Bifidobacterium can be found in breast milk. As such, it is not surprising that Bifidobacterium can be detected in feces within two days of birth and is known to colonize in almost all infants by the end of their first week of life. Shortly after, Bifidobacterium will dominate the infant's microflora, as long as breast-feeding continues.

Probiotics are slower to colonize in infants who are fed infant formulas than infants who are breast-fed, as breast milk has oligosaccharides, a prebiotic that helps feed the probiotics in the baby. The reason that Bifidobacteria appears to be the most dominant microbe in infants is probably because there is always lots of their preferred food source, oligosaccharides, available in breast milk.

When probiotics are slow to colonize in an infant's intesti-

| *Abnormal gut microflora at an early age may predispose you to disease later in life.*

nal tract, it allows bad bacteria to enter the infant's system. This is a concern for premature babies that require intensive care. If colonization is irregular in a premature infant's gut, it may increase their risk of develping necrotizing enterocolitis (death of the intestinal lining). Probiotic supplementation may be of help. Probiotics help inhibit the growth of bad microbes in infants, increasing their risk of developing a normal, healthy microflora. Many experts believe that the presence of bad microbes in an infant's intestinal tract may increase their risk of disease later in life.

Starting at weaning, the microflora in an infant grows more complex and offers more health benefits to the body; however, the diversity and activity of microbes seen in adults may not be seen in a child for several years after weaning.

WHAT TYPE OF BACTERIA LIVE IN INFANTS?

Which probiotics are present in an infant's intestinal tract? Surprisingly, Lactobacilli account for less than 1% of the total microflora in infants. Yet Bifidobacteria make up 60% to 90% of the microbes found in the feces of breast-fed infants. Original studies found *Bifidobacterium breve* and *Bifidobacterium bifidum* are the most common species in healthy infants. More recent studies have identified *Bifidobacterium infantis*, *Bifidobacterium longum* and *Bifidobacterium breve* as the species most often found in infants. In addition, *Bifidobacterium animalis* and *Bifidobacterium catenulatum* were reportedly found frequently in infants tested in a 2007 study. These probiotics are introduced to an infant from breast milk. Their exact health benefits are not yet known.

The greatest difference between breast-fed and formula-fed infants appears to be a difference in how quickly and what types of probiotics colonize in the gut. In breast-fed infants, *Lactobacillus gasseri* was at first thought to be the most common Lactobacilli species. Yet more recent studies have shown that the *Lactobacillus acidophilus* is the most common Lactobacilli in both breast-fed and formula-fed infants. Infants consuming infant formula are known to have fewer types of species and quantity of Bifidiobacteria. Some newer infant formulas developed after the turn of the century now include probiotics and prebiotics, as the presence of probiotics early in an infant's life is recognized as having great importance in newborn health. If your child is using infant formula that does not include a probiotic or contain any prebiotics, supplements can be added to his or her formula which contain the main Bifidobacteria species known to live in healthy infants.

PREBIOTICS FOR INFANTS?

As an infant's microflora is dominated by Bifidobacteria, prebiotics are thought to benefit the development of a healthy microflora in infants. Bifidobacteria are stimulated by prebiotics and as such, it is not surprising that breast milk is naturally high in prebiotics. Do we know if prebiotic supplementation can benefit the health of infants? Researchers investigated the effects of an oligofructose ingredient (a prebiotic) in a group of 35 infants (6 to 24 months of age), who were attending a daycare center in Paris, France. The researchers found that the children supplemented with the prebiotic had positive changes to their microflora and showed improvements in their overall well-being. Thus, prebiotics such as inulin and oligofructose are thought to play a helpful role in promoting health in infants and should be an ingredient of infant formulas.

WHICH PROBIOTIC SPECIES IS MOST IMPORTANT TO INFANT HEALTH?

Certain Bifidobacteria species are known to live in healthy infants, but what other species are important is not yet known. Changes in intestinal microflora may increase an infant's risk of developing allergic diseases. A decrease in the number of Bifidobacteria, or an increase in number of bad microbes, e.g., Clostridium, are examples of changes in the microflora that can increase an infant's risk of developing allergic diseases. Luckily, research has discovered that certain probiotic species can prevent such changes in microflora and reduce illness in infants.

Probiotics were first used to prevent infant disease in a clinical trial in 1994. In the randomized trial held in Baltimore, 55 infants were given an infant formula with or without *Bifidobacterium bifidum* and *Streptococcus thermophilus*. Infants are commonly infected with Rotavirus, the most frequent cause of diarrhea in children. These probiotics significantly reduced the risk of diarrhea and the growth of Rotavirus. Diarrhea only occurred in 7% of the infants receiving probiotics; meanwhile, 31% of the controls developed diarrhea. *B. bifidum* and *S. thermophilus* were successful in preventing illness in these infants. These two species of probiotics may be good additions to infant formulas.

Another probiotic, *Lactobacillus rhamnosus* GG may also prevent diarrhea. Four clinical trials have given *Lactobacillus rhamnosus* GG to infants and the results suggest it can help prevent diarrhea. More research is needed before this species gains the title of "diarrhea-preventor." *Lactobacillus reuteri* and *Bifidobacteria lactis* are two other probiotic species that have shown excellent results in clinical trials and are good choices for a child with diarrhea. Many research papers have supported the use of probiotics in infants as a safe and effective way to treat diarrhea.

The ability of probiotics to prevent illness in infants goes beyond diarrhea. In 2005, a large study investigated the effects of probiotics on the health of children in childcare centres. The study included 14 childcare centers across Israel. Healthy infants between four and 10 months of age were either given their regular formula, or a formula supplemented with *Bifidobacterium lactis* or *Lactobacillus reuteri*. The chidren receiving probiotics did not get sick as often as the children who were not supplemented. The children receiving *L. reuteri* were the least sick. In other words, *L. reuteri* appears to prevent illness best in children, compared to *B. lactis* or placebo. According to this study, supplementing with *L. reuteri* significantly decreases the number of days infants have a fever, need to visit a clinic, are absent from child care and need to use antibiotics. The bifidus species *B. lactis* also decreased how frequently the children were sick. *B. lactis* and *L. reuteri* can prevent illness in children. From this study we also know that probiotics can be useful in improving immunity and reducing the frequency of fever and bacterial illness in infants as young as four months of age.

Another study found that probiotics may reduce respiratory infections in children. *L. rhamnosus* GG has been shown to reduce the number of respiratory illnesses in children. Other studies are looking into whether there is the potential to treat and prevent respiratory problems in children with probiotic supplementation.

Probiotics can improve immunity in children.

It appears that probiotics help keep infants healthy. Probiotics are known to effect the maturation of the immune system, which is likely why in many studies probiotics are found to prevent infants from getting sick.

PROBIOTICS AND COLIC

Colic is another condition of infants that can be relieved with the use of probiotics. Colic is one of the most common problems during the first three months of an infant's life and can affect up to 28% of newborns. When the microflora of infants who are colicky and non-colicky are compared, the infants suffering from colic tend to have fewer Lactobacilli probiotics in their intestines and more bad microbes. A study done by researchers at the University of Turin found that probiotics could reduce the crying time of infants with colic by 75%. The probiotic species used was *L. reuteri,* and it improved colicky symptoms in breast-fed infants within one week of treatment. Probiotics were tested against the pharmaceutical simethicone and were found to be significantly better at making colicky infants happier. This suggests that probiotics have a role to play in treating colic.

SUMMARY

Adult humans have over 400 species of microflora living in their intestinal tract, yet at birth an infant's intestinal tract is almost sterile. It only takes minutes for microbes to invade a newborn's body. The first microbes in an infant's body are the mother's. A mother's microflora can affect labor time and influence the makeup of an infant's microflora. Breast-feeding appears to promote the presence of healthy microflora in newborn infants. Bifidobacteria are the dominant species in infants with *B. breve, B. infantis, B. longum* and *B. bifidum* being the dominant species. Some Lactobacilli are present in an infant's microflora, but not at levels seen in adults. Despite the difference in composition, probiotics appear to offer an infant similar health benefits as seen in adults. Probiotics improve immunity and prevent diarrhea according to clinical research. Probiotics likely play a role in colic and *L. reuteri* is known to reduce crying times in these infants. Probiotics may reduce the risk of children developing allergic diseases later in life and may play a role in reducing respiratory-related illnesses. Research to date has found supplementing probiotics in infant formulas to be safe and effective in infants as young as four months of age. Prebiotics may be of particular benefit to infants as their microflora is predominantly Bifidobacteria.

c h a p t e r
8

Probiotic Rescue: Intestinal Dysbiosis, Irritable Bowel Syndrome and Inflammatory Bowel Disease

A MICROSCOPIC VIEW OF THIS CHAPTER

- The type and number of probiotics in the intestines affects health.
- Negative changes in intestinal microflora is called *dysbiosis*.
- Dysbiosis may cause many diseases, including inflammatory bowel diseases.
- Probiotics aid intestinal disorders.
- People with irritable bowel syndrome may benefit from probiotics.
- Probiotics promote intestinal health.
- Inflammatory bowel diseases include ulcerative colitis and Crohn's disease.
- Inflammation causing damage in these diseases can be reduced by probiotics.
- Prebiotics and the use of multiple species of probiotics can rescue the intestines.

■ ■ ■ ■ ■ ■ ■

The gastrointestinal tract is one of the largest points of contact between the outside world and your internal environment. From your mouth to anus, the gastrointestinal tract forms a 30-foot-long tube.

In fact, your gastrointestinal tract is your body's second-largest surface area, the first being the skin.

The gastrointestinal tract is the body's second-largest surface area.

Over a normal lifetime, about 60 tons of food will pass through your gastrointestinal tract. Everyone agrees that food is extremely important for well-being; however, its passage through your gastrointestinal tract is actually a threat to your health. Yes, food provides nutrients vital to your health, yet in digesting and absorbing these nutrients, food exposes you to antigens, bad microbes and toxic chemicals. As the second-largest surface area in the body, the gastrointestinal tract is a big area through which harmful things try to gain access into your body.

THE MICROFLORA AND INTESTINAL DISEASES

Probiotic research studies have been published in a wide variety of scientific journals including those focusing on pediatrics, gastrointestinal health, pharmaceuticals and nutrition. Probiotic research involves an unusually wide range of disciplines: pediatrics, gastroenterology, nutrition, immunology and microbiology. This is what makes this new area of health so fascinating—it affects your entire body at every stage of life! Some of the most promising areas of research on probiotics relates to inflammatory intestinal disorders. These diseases affect many and no cure has yet been found.

Why are probiotics so promising in the field of intestinal health? Consider the following. Intestinal microbes outnumber cells in the human body 10-fold. The microflora of your body has a metabolic activity that is the same as your organs. The microflora is kind of a virtual organ, sometimes called the "neglected organ." Thus, the type and number of intestinal microbes have a great impact on our intestinal tract's health, immune response and may be involved in many intestinal disease conditions.

The intestinal tract is lined with a mucus layer that is produced by the intestinal cells. The normal flora in the intestinal tract has an important influence on the structure, function and development of the mucus layer. Probiotics and bad microbes interact with these cells affecting the mucus layer and the body's response to things that stimulate inflammation, e.g., bad microbes and allergens. Probiotics and bad microbes also exchange signals with the immune system that lies below the intestinal lining. Since probiotics can talk with your immune system, they are able to help reduce inflammation-related illnesses such as irritable bowel disease.

Diseases of the intestinal tract commonly involve inflammation. Irritable bowel syndrome (IBS), inflammatory bowel disease (IBD), Crohn's disease, ulcerative colitis, intestinal dysbiosis and pouchitis all involve the immune system. Because probiotics can talk with the immune system in the intestinal tract, scientists think that probiotics can help rescue you from these disease conditions.

There are more bacteria in the gut than cells in the body.

INTESTINAL DYSBIOSIS

Repeatedly we see the importance of a balanced, healthy microflora in the intestinal tract. When this balance is altered, intestinal **dysbiosis** (a negative change in the intestinal microflora) occurs and numerous diseases can result. An imbalance in the intestinal flora can be caused by a number of factors associated with modern Western living. Factors such as antibiotics, psychological and physical stress, chronic diarrhea or constipation and certain foods have been found to contribute to intestinal dysbiosis. Intestinal dysbiosis has symptoms that include bloating, flatulence, abdominal pain, diarrhea and/ or constipation. This imbalance in intestinal flora can lead to fungal overgrowth, e.g., Candida. Yeast infections can cause itchiness, redness, heat and pain.

Dysbiosis

The term *dysbiosis* was originally coined by Metchnikoff to describe a change in bad microbes in the gut. Today, dysbiosis is described as a state in which the microflora produces harmful effects via: (1) changes in the number and type of intestinal flora; (2) changes in their metabolic activities; and (3) changes in their local distribution.

Our modern diet and lifestyle, and use of antibiotics can lead to a disruption of our normal intestinal microflora. These factors cause unfavorable changes in the growth of probiotics and bad microbes and can increase the amount of toxic products in your gut, all of which play a role in many chronic and degenerative diseases, including irritable bowel syndrome, inflammatory bowel disease (e.g., colitis and Crohn's disease) and systemic conditions such as rheumatoid arthritis. This is called the *dysbiosis hypothesis.*

The intestinal mucosa is the mucus coating in the gastrointestinal tract. It plays a dual role: absorbing nutrients and stopping bad substances from getting into the body (through the bloodstream). The health and strength of the intestinal mucosa are very important to immunity and health. The food we consume exposes the gastrointestinal tract to bad microbes that can produce ammonia, endotoxins, hydrogen sulphide, phenols and indoles. These toxic products can have detrimental effects on both the mucus lining of your intestines and the health of your body. The amount of these toxins present in your intestinal tract is dependent on the nutrients you eat and the type of microbes in your intestinal tract. To explain, diets that are high in protein and sulfates (a food additive) have been shown to promote the production of these toxins by bad microbes in your intestinal tract. In other words, avoiding these foods and keeping your probiotics healthy are great ways to reduce these toxins in your gut.

Prebiotics are another food you can eat that will affect the health of your intestinal mucus lining and your intestinal cells. Prebiotics selectively promote probiotics, helping them grow in your intestines. Since probiotics can fight bad microbes and promote the health of your intestinal cells and mucus lining, prebiotics are an important food to add to your diet.

The theory that intestinal dysbiosis causes so many diseases of the intestinal tract has created a deep appreciation for the effect your microflora has on your health. You need to maintain a healthy balance of microflora in your intestinal tract to enjoy health. Probiotics, prebiotics and a proper diet can help.

Changes in the natural intestinal microflora can lead to chronic and degenerative diseases.

Alterations in intestinal flora are thought to play a role in many gastrointestinal disease conditions including irritable bowel syndrome, inflammatory bowel disease (e.g., colitis and Crohn's disease) and systemic conditions such as rheumatoid arthritis. Research has found probiotics play a protective and beneficial role in these disease conditions. Let's discover what we know to date about these diseases and probiotics.

IRRITABLE BOWEL SYNDROME

About 20 percent of adults have irritable bowel syndrome (IBS). It is one of the most common syndromes diagnosed by doctors. It occurs more often in women than in men, and it begins before the age of 35 in about 50% of people. By definition, irritable bowel syndrome is "a functional gastrointestinal disorder that includes a combination of chronic or recurrent gastrointestinal symptoms that cannot be explained by structural or biochemical abnormalities."

Irritable bowel syndrome is characterized by abdominal pain, excessive gas, bloating and changes in intestinal movement and transit. There is no evidence of detectable organic disease. The main symptom criterion is abdominal pain that is relieved by going to the bathroom (defecation) or that is associated with changes in frequency or consistency of stools.

Gastroenteritis and antibiotic use are currently thought to be environmental risk factors for developing irritable bowel syndrome. *Irritable bowel syndrome is reported as the leading cause of work absenteeism, second only to the common cold.* Researchers have noted a link between the onset of irritable bowel syndrome and a recent episode of gastroenteritis where the person used antibiotics. Inflammation disturbs the natural reflexes or movements of the intestinal tract, according to human and animal studies. Also, inflammation activates the **visceral sensory system** even if the inflammatory response is minimal. Research suggests that a change in your intestinal microflora may be an underlying cause (**etiology** factor) of irritable bowel syndrome.

Naturally, researchers have wondered if probiotic therapy could be a preventative or potential treatment for irritable bowel syndrome. From the first research study investigating probiotics in patients with irritable bowel syndrome there has been excitement about the potential for this therapy. Some probiotics exhibit antibacterial, anti-viral and anti-inflammatory properties and can restore the intestinal microflora balance, suggesting that they may become a treatment for irritable bowel syndrome.

The earliest reported use of probiotics to treat gastrointestinal concerns was in 1955, when Winkelstein compiled a series of case studies from his private practice. He reported resolving constipation or diarrhea problems in 26 patients with daily administration of an unidentified strain of *Lactobacillus acidophilus*. Unfortunately, it was not until the 1980s that controlled trials were reported.

Lactobacillus acidophilus LB was used in the first controlled trial and was found to significantly reduce symptoms of irritable bowel syndrome. Many other species of probiotics have been used in con-trolled trials to treat irritable bowel syndrome. Here is a summary of the findings of the effects of various probiotic species on irritable bowel syndrome.

L. acidophilus and L. rhamnosus

Clinical studies have found modest improvements in irritable bowel syndrome symptoms with *Lactobacillus acidophilus* supplementation. A combination of *L. acidophilus* and *L. rhamnosus* has beneficial ef-fects on irritable bowel symptoms.

L. paracasei

Research suggests that *Lactobacillus paracasei* NCC2461 appears to help reduce inflammation and improves movement in the bowels of those suffering from irritable bowel syndrome.

L. plantarum

L. plantarum has consistently produced improvement in patients with irritable bowel syndrome in clinical studies. For example, a European study in 2001 found *L. plantarum* reduced all irritable bowel syndrome symptoms in 95% of patients after four weeks of supplementation. Another study gave *L. plantarum* for four weeks to 60 people with irritable bowel syndrome. This double-blind, placebo-controlled trial found that one year after the study, people who received the probiotic reported significant reductions in flatulence and maintained a better overall intestinal function.

B. infantis

A team from the Alimentary Pharmabiotic Centre at Ireland's University College Cork reported that irritable bowel syndrome patients who consumed a *Bifidobacterium infantis* drink every day for eight weeks experienced fewer overall symptoms, abdominal pain and discomfort. At the American College of Gastroenterology meeting in 2005, a study was presented that showed *Bifidobacterium infantis* significantly reduced symptoms of irritable bowel syndrome in 165 women in four weeks. The probiotic was able to normalize bowel movements in the women who had either constipation or diarrhea. These results are the same as previous results in which *Bifidobacterium infantis* taken daily for eight weeks reduced overall irritable bowel syndrome symptoms, abdominal pain and discomfort. The relief experienced with probiotic supplementation is similar to that seen with the approved irritable bowel syndrome pharmaceuticals Zelnorm (tegaserod) and Lotronex (alosetron).

L. salivarius

L. salivarius may help people with irritable bowel syndrome. In an eight-week double-blind, placebo-controlled trial *L. salivarius* was found to be superior in causing improvements in patients to *B. infantis*.

B. lactis

Bifidiobacteria lactis 35624 appears to alleviate irritable bowel symptoms and affect inflammation. This probiotic species positively changes the ratio of good to bad inflammatory chemicals (e.g., IL-10 to IL-12), promoting healthy inflammation in the intestines.

Safety in IBS

The use of probiotics in people suffering from irritable bowel syndrome has been very successful and presents no safety concerns. As this therapy is also inexpensive compared to pharmaceutical alternatives, probiotics hold promise as a future therapy for irritable bowel syndrome patients.

Prebiotics and IBS

Prebiotics may also offer some help to those suffering from irritable bowel syndrome. A number of studies have looked at the ability of prebiotics to improve symptoms in those suffering from irritable bowel syndrome—the results are promising. In particular, prebiotics offer a safe way to improve health in those suffering from irritable bowel syndrome–related constipation.

Probiotics for the treatment of irritable bowel syndrome has shown promising results in clinical trials. Over two dozen trials have attempted to address this issue. Few trials that compare probiotic species or use combinations of species have been conducted to date to help us make a conclusive recommendation of which species will offer the best effects for those with irritable bowel syndrome. However, many species have been shown in clinical trials to offer benefits to those with irritable bowel syndrome. As such, one can assume that supplementation with a diversity of probiotics that are known to be beneficial can offer the best health benefits to irritable bowel syndrome patients. The use of probiotics has resulted in improvements in irritable bowel symptoms in many studies and clinical case reports. The therapy is safe and relatively inexpensive. Prebiotics should also be considered in an irritable bowel syndrome treatment plan.

INFLAMMATORY BOWEL DISEASE

It is estimated that two million people worldwide are affected by inflammatory bowel disease (IBD). Inflammatory bowel disease is the name of a group of disorders that cause the intestines to become inflamed. There are two clinical **phenotypes** of inflammatory bowel disease: ulcerative colitis and Crohn's disease. Both include inflammation in the intestine. In ulcerative colitis, the inflammation is limited to the colon. In Crohn's disease, inflammation may also be present in the small intestine. Symptoms of inflammatory bowel disease involve disruption in bowel habits and mucosal inflammation. It is thought to be caused by environmental substances, including your diet and intestinal microflora. Disturbance of intestinal microflora, i.e., dysbiosis, is a key factor causing inflammatory bowel disease.

To what degree the environment causes inflammatory bowel disease is uncertain. However, if environmental causes of inflammatory bowel disease can be eliminated, then treatments to help rebuild a healthy microflora may be very successful. As such, dietary changes, probiotics and prebiotics could be very successful treatments for inflammatory bowel disease if it is caused by an unhealthy microflora (intestinal dysbiosis). Reducing the intake of proteins and processed foods, particularly those containing sulfates, can help reduce fermentation that results in the creation of some toxic compounds (ammonia, endotoxins) in the gastrointestinal tract. Another way to reduce the production of toxic compounds in the gastrointestinal tract is to ensure probiotics are present. Probiotics have positive effects that increase the ability of the intestinal mucosa's to filter out toxins, preventing them from getting into your blood. You can increase the amount of probiotics in your intestine by supplementing with them or eating foods that contain prebiotics that promote the growth of probiotics. Prebiotics are dietary components used to fight dysbiosis. Prebiotics can selectively promote probiotics, a perfect way to fight dysbiosis.

The **etiology** of inflammatory bowel disease likely involves three factors:

The development of irritable bowel disease may be caused by an intolerance to normal microbes by the immune system.

- your susceptibility
- the health of your intestinal mucus lining
- your current level of probiotics.

There are many theories as to the cause of inflammatory bowel disease; however, a growing number of experts are giving the intestinal microflora a second look. Research in both animals and humans with inflammatory bowel disease suggest that the microflora is one of the factors involved in the tissue damage seen in this disease. In susceptible individuals, inflammatory bowel disease may arise due to a breakdown in their immune system, which does not tolerate the microbes that live in their intestine and reacts to them as if they were not helpful, but harmful. The drugs that are used today to treat irritable bowel disease try to reduce the ability of your immune system to attack the microbes in your intestines, thus relieving some of the symptoms, but this also reduces your ability to fight disease in other parts of your body. These drugs suppress your immune system, making it easier for you to get sick. Using probiotics and prebiotics to help change the type of microbes in your intestines might stop the immune system from attacking and reducing the irritable bowel disease symptoms. Probiotics and prebiotics may be a good option to try when using drugs, as they may help reduce symptoms of the disease and can help protect you while your immune system is weak.

Research to date has shown that probiotics do not cure inflammatory bowel disease. Yet probiotics do significantly prolong remission, which can increase your quality of life. By changing the intestinal flora with the use of probiotics and prebiotics you may be able to reduce the symptoms of irritable bowel disease.

CROHN'S DISEASE

What is Crohn's disease? Crohn's disease is a chronic inflammatory disease involving the small and large intestine, but which can affect other parts of the digestive system as well. It is named for Burrill Crohn, the American gastroenterologist who first described the disease in 1932. Crohn's disease is usually diagnosed in people in their teens or 20s, but can be diagnosed at any point in life. It can be a chronic, recurring condition, or it can cause minimal symptoms with or without medical treatment, depending on the person.

What is the relationship between microbes and Crohn's disease? This relationship is not completely understood. Researchers have discovered that some strains of *Escherichia coli,* a bad microbe, may be involved in Crohn's disease. Other microbes are thought to be beneficial and protective to the intestinal tract: Bifidobacteria and Lactobacilli.

Several randomized control trials have looked at the ability of probiotics to help people with Crohn's disease. The evidence strongly supports the use of probiotics in those suffering from Crohn's disease. Both Lactobacilli and Bifidobacteria have been shown to support a healthy intestinal tract and reduce problems with Crohn's disease. This makes sense that both families of probiotics are helpful, if you remember that Crohn's disease infects both the small intestinal tract and the colon (the two locations where these probiotics love to live).

Some promising results have been seen when the probiotic *Lactobacillus rhamnosus* GG was used in combination with immunomodulatory drugs such as Prednisone in people with Crohn's disease. The study found an improvement in symptoms in one week. There also appeared to be an improvement in the health of the gut barrier. This means that fewer bad microbes or allergens were able to irritate the intestines.

Other probiotics including *L. salivarius* and *Saccharomyces boulardii* have shown promising preliminary results in Crohn's disease studies and may be helpful in promoting general intestinal health. In fact, both lactic acid bacteria *L. rhamnosus* GG and *L. salivarius* UCC 118, as well as *Escherichia coli* Nissle are currently thought to be effective in maintaining remission of inflammatory bowel disease.

Lactobacillus plantarum may also offer some help to intestinal tracts plagued by inflammatory diseases such as Crohn's disease. Critically ill, antibiotic-treated inflammatory bowel disease patients were supplemented with *L. plantarum*. The probiotic was able to live in the colon, where it reduced the number of bad microbes (enterobacteriacea). This is helpful as fewer bad microbes mean less toxins to irritate the colon and cause symptoms. Daily use of *L. plantarum* may offer some help in critically ill, antibiotic-treated inflammatory bowel disease patients.

Bifidobacterium, which mostly live in the colon, are also thought to be of help for Crohn's disease sufferers. Research has investigated Bifidobacterium species (*B. breve, B. infantis, B. longum*) and found they may have a beneficial effect by controlling immune factors, called *cytokine transcription factors*, within the mucus of the intestines. In Crohn's disease it is the inflammation that causes the symptoms—less inflammation means happier intestines. Bifidobacterium also appears to help control immune cells in the intestinal mucus, which are called *T cells*. By controlling the inflammation in the intestinal mucus, Bifidobacteria may be able to reduce symptoms and problems associated with inflammatory bowel diseases like Crohn's disease. Bifidobacteria are a promising Crohn's disease therapy.

Both Lactobacilli and Bifidobacteria species are helpful in those with Crohn's disease. How about a combination of two probiotic families? A combination probiotic called VSL#3, which includes *L. casei, L. plantarum, L. acidophilus, L. bulgaricus, B. longum, B. breve, B. infantis, S. thermophilus, E. coli* Nissle 1917 and *S. boulardii*, has also shown positive results in alleviating symptoms of inflammatory bowel disease. Many different probiotics are known to be helpful for those with Crohn's disease.

> **A Unique Prebiotic for IBD**
>
> Interesting research on germinated barley foodstuff (GBF) was published in 2000. GBF is a prebiotic whose unique characteristics make it highly suitable for applications in irritable bowel disease. GBF is converted in the body by probiotics of the Eubacterium and Bifidobacterium genus into butyrate, which causes anti-inflammtory effects in the intestines and accelerates intestinal epithelial cell growth, i.e., helps the intestinal lining heal quickly.

Prebiotics may also offer some help for people with Crohn's disease. Prebiotics help feed probiotics in the intestintal tract, improving their numbers. As such, prebiotics may be a good addition to the diet of people with Crohn's disease as healthy populations of probiotics is known to help them feel better.

PROBIOTIC ROCKETS FOR TREATMENT

The next stage in inflammatory bowel disease research may involve genetically modified probiotics. We can send humans to the moon in rockets. Soon we may also be able to send treatments to the gut in probiotics. Probiotics can be the rocket for treatments. Advances in technology are trying to create organisms that can cure disease. Probiotics can be altered into genetically modified organisms that can deliver important substances to the intestines to help fight disease.

Let's explain how this might work. Crohn's disease involves many chemicals that promote inflammation. Some chemicals in the body can stop inflammation. Interleukin-10 (IL-10) is an inflammatory chemical that can stop inflammation and reduce symptoms of Crohn's disease and other inflammatory bowel diseases. Researchers have been able to genetically engineer *Lactococcus lactis* to deliver IL-10. The *L. lactis* was altered by researchers to be able to deliver interleukin-10 in the gut to help reduce inflammation there. It was tested in the **lumen** of mice with inflammatory bowel disease. *L. lactis* is a good probiotic to choose as it does not cause disease, is non-invasive and does not colonize in the body, so it cannot grow and create more IL-10. *L. lactis* has been safely used for years in the production of fermented foods. In this experiment, after two weeks of use, the probiotic significantly reduced the inflammation in the intestines. Perhaps future advances in this technology will allow us to cure Crohn's disease and other inflammatory bowel diseases with the help of this and other genetically modified probiotics.

ULCERATIVE COLITIS

Ulcerative colitis is a type of inflammatory bowel disease that affects the large intestine and rectum. The cause of this disease is unknown. It may affect any age group, although its occurence peaks at ages 15 to 30 and then again at ages 50 to 70. The disease usually begins in the rectal area and may eventually extend through the entire large intestine. The disease causes inflammation to the intestinal wall. Repeated inflammation causes the wall to thicken and scar tissue to develop. The tissue of the colon can even die or become infected with bacteria in severe cases of the disease.

Ulcerative colitis is a chronic disease with frequent relapses. In humans with ulcerative colitis, the inflammation occurs where there is the highest bacterial concentration—the colon and rectum. The usual therapy for ulcerative colitis is a combination of drugs called *sulfasalazine* and *glucocorticosteroids*. The aim and hope of this therapy is to stop the inflammation and keep the person in a state of remission. However, a large number of patients become resistant or intolerant to sulfasalazine, and this treatment no longer offers help.

Probiotics can also cause remission of ulcerative colitis. A number of trials have found single probiotic strains to help improve health in people with inflammatory bowel disease such as ulcerative colitis. Probiotics are well supported as a way to help people with this disease.

What about using multiple species to treat ulcerative colitis? In a clinical trial, a probiotic mixture including four strains of Lactobacilli, three strains of Bifidobacteria and *Streptococcus thermophilus* was given to a number of ulcerative colitis patients. This high dosage, multi-strain probiotic mixture improved the number of patients and duration of their remission, and decreased inflammation.

A review of all of the clinical research on the use of probiotics in people with ulcerative colitis suggests that high-dose, multi-strain probiotic mixtures are more effective at reducing inflammation and increasing remission length than single probiotic strains. Of note, the probiotic *Escherichia coli* has also been used in a number of clinical trials and reportedly maintains remission in ulcerative colitis patients.

POUCHITIS

Patients with ulcerative colitis sometimes have part of their colon removed to treat the disease. In this surgery, physicians will sometimes create an internal pouch, called an *ileoanal pouch*, to prevent the need to wear an external appliance to store stool (fecal waste). Sometimes the lining of this internal pouch becomes inflamed. This complication is known as pouchitis. Thirty-two percent of patients with an ileoanal pouch have had at least one episode of pouchitis. Pouchitis can cause symptoms similar to ulcerative colitis, such as crampy abdominal pain, diarrhea, dehydration, increased frequency of stool, fever, bleeding and joint pain. Typically, pouchitis is treated with the short-term use of antibiotics. Antibiotics are generally effective at reducing inflammation and promoting remission in these people. However, there are side effects of using antibiotics. including an increased risk of diarrhea and an increased risk of complications in the intestines due to the loss of probiotics.

Probiotics are leading the way for a new treatment option for pouchitis. Probiotics not only promote remission of pouchitis, they also appear to have preventative effects. Clinical trials have found that probiotics have the ability to maintain remission in patients suffering from recurrent pouchitis. A number of randomized, placebo-controlled trials involving patients with recent remission from pouchitis due to antibiotic use have found that probiotics can help maintain remission for at least a year.

It appears that supplementing with probiotics of multiple species has a greater positive effect on pouchitis than taking only a single species. A high dosage of a probiotic mixture including four different strains of Lactobacillus, three Bifidobacteria strains and *Streptococcus thermophilus* was used in a randomized, placebo-controlled study and found to be effective at maintaining antibiotic-induced remission in patients with pouchitis. The probiotic treatment also reduced the likelihood of relapse.

Another popular multi-strain probiotic combination called VSL#3 has been found to be effective against pouchitis remisison. VSL#3 is a combination of *L. casei, L. plantarum, L. acidophilus, L. bulgaricus, B. longum, B. breve, B. infantis* and *S. thermophilus*. In a large clinical trial, volunteers were given pharmaceuticals to induce remission of their pouchitis and then randomly given either VSL#3 or placebo. Of the patients getting no probiotics, 100% experienced relapse. Only 15% of the patients taking probiotics experienced relapses of pouchitis. Probiotics can decrease the likelihood of relapse in patients in remission of pouchitis.

On the contrary, research investigating the effects of a single probiotic, *Lactobacillus rhamnosus* GG, did not show a clinical effect on pouchitis. Perhaps this particular strain is not helpful or the symptoms of pouchitis can only be helped by the presence of multiple probiotic species.

When all of the scientific literature is considered, it is easy to conclude that there is an advantage to taking several probiotic strains at high doses to treat pouchitis. Researchers also suggest that probiotics may reduce the risk of developing pouchitis in patients undergoing ulcerative colitis surgery.

Of note, probiotics are not effective in inducing remission from pouchitis. Remission can be induced by antibiotic use. Clinical trials have shown that remission can be effectively maintained with probiotic use. Many studies have reported that both probiotics and antibiotics can be used at the same time, and this is a safe and effective means of treatment in many disease conditions. Of note, they should be taken a few hours apart to avoid interaction. The use of both may offer the best solution to patients with pouchitis.

SUMMARY

Probiotics love to live in the intestinal tract, where they offer many healthy benefits to all of us. Changes in the number and type of microbes in the intestines have many negative affects on your health. One of the most common health problems in Western civilization is inflammation in the intestines. This can cause a wide array of symptoms.

Irritable bowel syndrome is a term used to explain chronic unhealthy and unhappy symptoms in the intestines. There is no known cause of this illness. Probiotics have been found to improve the health of those suffering from irritable bowel syndrome. Many species are known to reduce symptoms and a combination of a number of these species is currently thought to offer the most help to people with irritable bowel syndrome. Prebiotics may also be helpful.

A large body of evidence suggests that your intestinal microflora is a factor in inflammatory diseases of the intestinal tract. Inflammation in the intestinal tract can become chronic. Inflammatory bowel diseases include Crohn's disease, irritable bowel disease and ulcerative colitis. People with irritable bowel disease seem to have unusual microbe populations in their intestines. This suggests that changing the type and quantity of probiotics in the intestines likely will help those with irritable bowel disease.

Crohn's disease is a chronic inflammatory disease that affects both the small and large intestine. Both Lactobacillus and Bifidobacterium species have been found in clinical studies to effectively benefit individuals with inflammatory bowel disease. Single strains appear to have beneficial effects as do multi-strain probiotic combinations. No one strain is known to be the best; however, it appears that a combination of Lactobacilli and Bifidobacteria is ideal as these species love to live in both areas of the intestines affected by these diseases.

The use of probiotics as an extra therapy for inflammatory bowel diseases has been well studied. These studies suggest that high doses of multi-species probiotics are effective in decreasing inflammation in people with inflammatory bowel disease.

Pouchitis, a complication experienced in patients with an ileoanal pouch, can maintain remission with probiotics. The use of probiotics at the same time as antibiotics may be of benefit to patients with pouchitis. High-dosage, multi-strain products appear to be the best choice for those with pouchitis.

Prebiotics help make positive changes to the microflora in the intestines. As such, prebiotics are thought to help with many of these diseases of the intestinal tract. Those with inflammatory bowel diseases should consider adding prebiotics to their diet or taking them as supplements to help improve their intestinal health.

chapter

9

Allergies and Probiotics

A MICROSCOPIC VIEW OF THIS CHAPTER

- The intestinal microflora plays a role in immune system regulation.
- Probiotics promote healthy intestinal barriers and immune reactions.
- Lack of probiotics in infants may prevent proper immune maturation leading to allergies.
- Leaky gut allows allergens through the intestines and promotes allergies.
- Probiotics appear to prevent and treat certain *atopic diseases* (asthma, eczema).
- Eczema can be effectively treated with probiotics.
- Asthma may be prevented or treated with probiotics.
- Probiotics may play a role in food allergies.

■ ■ ■ ■ ■ ■ ■

What is an allergy? An allergy is an inappropriate immune reaction. In other words, the body is overreacting to an allergen (a substance that the body thinks is bad and defends itself against). Classic allergies are called type I hypersensitivity. In a classic allergy:

- An allergen enters the body.
- It interacts with immune cells called *mast cells*.
- The result is inflammation.

The inflammation can come in the form of itchy eyes, runny nose or diarrhea, depending on the allergen's route of entry. Chronic allergies commonly present themselves as asthma or eczema, which are called *atopic diseases*. **Atopic diseases** are allergic diseases that occur with exposure to a substance that someone is allergic too. In rare instances, an extreme reaction to an allergen can occur in the body; this is called ***anaphylactic shock*** and can result in death. This is an inappropriate reaction by the immune system.

Atopic Diseases

Atopic diseases such as eczema and asthma occur when the immune system is misbehaving, resulting in an allergic reaction, in the form of inflammation. Genetic and environmental factors are involved. Atopic diseases have a strong hereditary component: if both parents are affected by an atopic disease (or one parent and a sibling), 40% of offspring will be affected. The genetic influence is multifactorial—no single gene carries asthma or eczema. Children with affected parents are more likely to become sensitive to an allergen and to develop allergic inflammation.

The growing incidence of allergies in the Western world has brought great attention to atopic diseases. Atopic diseases include eczema, asthma and other allergies. Increased cleanliness and reduced exposure to microbes are thought to be involved in the growing number of allergies in the Western world. As probiotics are known to keep the immune system in check, researchers are focusing on the interaction between the intestinal microflora and the immune system. In fact, the intestinal microflora is not just good at keeping the immune system in line, it is an important factor in regulating both the intestinal immune system and the systemic (entire body) immune system.

| *Probiotics keep the immune system in check.*

Let's start at the beginning with infants. It is hypothesized that the increasing rate of allergies has occurred at the same time as the reduction in children's exposure to microbes. The use of infant formula and antibacterial cleaning products has reduced the exposure of probiotics and bad microbes to infants and may be a cause of the increased incidence of allergies we see today.

INFANT IMMUNITY AND ALLERGIES

The prevalence of atopic disease is steadily increasing in Western society. In fact, the increase has been so quick that it cannot be caused by genetics; there must be an environmental factor involved. Some scientists believe that the reason there are more allergies in Western society is due to our reduced exposure to microbes at an early age. This is called the *hygiene hypothesis.* Strict hygiene, smaller family sizes, better healthcare and sterile food, all restrict our exposure to microbes as infants. The hygiene hypothesis was suggested by David Strachan in 1989, as data was starting to show an increase in the number of people suffering from allergies. The Center for Disease Control and Prevention in the United States reported that the prevalence of asthma in the United States has doubled from approximately 6.8 million in 1978 to more than 15 million in 1998. In addition, about 5% of the U. S. population has asthma, an allergy-related disease, with the highest percentage being in children, five to 14 years of age. Allergies are a growing problem in our society.

An allergy is an exaggerated reaction by the body to a substance called an allergen. Allergens can be a substance that causes disease such as venom, or they can be a relatively safe substance such as pollen or even the body's own cells. To have an allergy, an individual is said to be sensitized to an allergen. There are many factors that are thought to increase your chances of becoming sensitized, including inflammation in your intestinal tract. An inflamed intestinal tract has wider gaps between cells, which allow allergens to access your body through your circulatory system and cause allergic reactions.

The atopic diseases (eczema and asthma) are the most common chronic diseases of childhood, affecting about one in four children in developed countries.

Inflammation of the intestinal tract can be regulated by probiotics. In fact, probiotics correct **lymphocyte** (white blood cell) imbalances. Probiotics are powerful stimulators of chemicals that control inflammation called *inflammatory mediators*, e.g., Th1 cytokines, IL-12 and IFN-gamma. Some species of Lactobacilli and Bifidobacilli improve the intestine's ability to process allergens that have been ingested in the diet. Thus, a healthy microflora in the intestinal tract is vital in regulating the immune response and in preventing and treating allergies.

Early exposure of the blood to allergens is thought to increase the likelihood of developing allergies; thus, reducing the ability of these allergens to gain access to your blood may be vital in reducing the prevalence of allergies. Probiotics can control intestinal inflammation and reduce any gaps through which allergens can gain access to your blood. In other words, probiotics can reduce the chance of having allergic reactions. Thus, it is possible that the presence of probiotics in infants can reduce the chance of them developing allergies.

Probiotics first enter a baby immediately after birth. Research has confirmed that the presence of probiotics in the intestine leads to the maturation of the immune system. The maturation of the immune system in many infants is reduced due to less exposure to probiotics; this is particularly true of those who are bottle fed. This lack of probiotic ingestion in bottle-fed infants is known to have consequences. In several studies infants who have atopic diseases tend to have increased *clostridia* (a bad microbe) and fewer Bifidobacteria in their stools, indicating an unhealthy intestinal microflora. Atopic disease in infants is associated with having an unhealthy or abnormal microflora.

Probiotics may prevent the development of allergies. A number of studies have investigated the effects of supplementing both expecting mothers and infants with probiotics. The research shows that probiotics play a role in allergy (atopic disease) development in children. Let's look at what research has found and which probiotic strains appear to be most effective against various forms of atopic diseases.

ATOPIC DERMATITIS

What is atopic dermatitis? Atopic dermatitis, or eczema, is a skin disease characterized by areas of severe itching, redness, scaling, and loss of the surface of the skin. Chronic presence of the rash results in thickening of the skin, as people will constantly scratch and rub at it. It is the most common of the many types of eczema.

Atopic dermatitis is frequently associated with other atopic (allergic) disorders, especially asthma and allergic rhinitis (hayfever). Atopic dermatitis is attributed to a dysfunction or problem with the immune system. This disease usually affects young children on the face, the elbows and knees. Older children and adults are usually affected on the sides of the neck and on the inside of the elbow and knee.

Atopic dermatitis is com- *The cost of atopic dermatitis in Canada is* monly seen in infants and *estimated to be $1.4 billion annually.* is thought to be related to the immune system. As the immune system is greatly affected by the microflora introduced at birth, scientists have questioned whether atopic dermatitis is associated with a lack of probiotic presence at a young age. Breast milk contains probiotics which support a healthy gastrointestinal tract in infants. The use of infant formulas reduces an infant's exposure to probiotics. As well, when a child is weaned from breast milk, his or her intake of probiotics drops. These two circumstances result in a decrease in intestinal probiotics and can allow bad microbes to enter the intestinal tract, colonize, cause inflammation and thus increase the potential for allergy development.

Probiotics Help Fight Atopic Disease

Studies support the use of probiotics in infants with atopic dermatitis as a means to reduce the symptoms of this painful condition. According to research from the University of Western Australia, probiotic supplementation with *L. fermentum* for four months significantly reduced atopic dermatitis in young children aged six to 18 months. Ninety-two percent of the children receiving the probiotics had improved by the 16th week, compared to only 63% of the control group.

Other studies agree with these findings. A double-blind, placebo-controlled, crossover study gave two Lactobacillus strains (*L. rhamnosus* and *L. reuteri*) in combinations for six weeks to children aged one to 13 years old. Over 50% of the children taking the probiotic combination experienced improvements in their eczema. Only 15% of the children in the control group felt their symptoms had improved. A combination of *L. rhamnosus* and *L. reuteri* appears to be beneficial in the management of atopic dermatitis. *L. reuteri* in particular has been tested in numerous trials and is known to help treat children with eczema, and it may have some potential as a means of prevention.

A third study is worth mentioning here. An infant formula containing *L. rhamnosus* GG and *B. lactis* Bb-12 reduced the symptoms of allergy more quickly than standard treatment of hydrolyzed infant formula in young children with atopic dermatitis in a clinical trial. The reduction in symptoms occurred after two months of probiotic supplementation. This was the first clinical trial to show that specific probiotic strains can modify allergic inflammation. What is most amazing about these studies is that they prove how probiotics not only affect the immune system in the intestines, but they also affect the inflammatory system in other areas of the body.

Probiotics not only affect the intestines but also affect the inflammatory system in other areas of the body. What effect might probiotic supplementation have in preventing atopic disease?

A group of Finnish researchers examined infants who had evidence of atopic eczema and were thought to have an increased risk of developing allergic disease. The infants were given a formula supplemented with a probiotic, *Bifidobacterium lactis*. The study included a control group who were given an infant formula that contained no additional probiotics. As with all studies, it is important to measure the effects. A compound found in the blood, called IgE, can be used to measure inflammation. Interestingly, the level or amount of bad microbes (*E. coli*) was related to the level of IgE in these infants. As such, the researchers think that bad microbes are involved in the development of an allergic response. How does this work? The bad microbes change the gastrointestinal environment by producing toxins and damaging intestinal cells. If the researchers are correct, then supplementing infant formula with probiotic bacteria may decrease and prevent allergic reactions.

Microscopic Heroes

Why would probiotics help? Probiotics alter the immune system to encourage the body's barriers to be strong, thereby reducing the ability of allergens to enter the blood or circulatory system. The inflammatory molecule IgA acts like a soldier that guards your intestines, preventing allergens from getting into your body. IgA acts as one of the first lines of defense against invaders. On the mucus surfaces of the body, such as those lining the gastrointestinal and respiratory tracts, IgA protects you from bad microbes and allergens that enter your body every time you breathe and ingest food. More specifically, IgA inhibits the ability of bad microbes to bind to the mucus surface of your body. Increasing the number of IgA molecules on the surface of the intestinal tract reduces the ability of bad microbes to attach and colonize.

The colonization of bad microbes in the intestinal tract can cause inflammation and is associated with allergy development. Thus, a way to increase IgA expression may help reduce the risk of developing an allergy. A study of infants with atopic dermatitis was conducted to see what effect probiotics have on IgA expression in the gastrointestinal tract. The study involved 230 infants who were given a placebo or a *Lactobacillus rhamnosus* GG milk mixture for four weeks. They found that the group consuming the probiotics had greater IgA secretion, suggesting that probiotics promote (upregulate) the defenses of the intestines. This research shows how probiotics beneficially alter inflammation and factors that promote allergy development.

Preventing Atopic Disease

Does this mean that probiotics can prevent the development of atopic dermatitis? At McMaster University in Canada, 1223 pregnant women carrying children at high-risk of developing atopic dermatitis were randomized to use a probiotic preparation or a placebo for two to four weeks before delivery. For sixth months after birth, their infants received the placebo or the same probiotics as their mother, plus galacto-oligosaccharides, a prebiotic. After two years, the incidence of allergic diseases (food allergy, eczema, asthma and allergic rhinitis) was evaluated. There were healthy amounts of Lactobacilli and Bifidobacterium species in the supplemented children. The children in the probiotic group had less atopic eczema. Probiotics can prevent eczema. The results suggest there is an inverse relationship between the presence of probiotics in an infant's intestinal tract and the development of atopic diseases. In other words, probiotics do appear to reduce atopic disease.

Another study found that the prevalence of atopic eczema can be reduced in half with probiotic supplementation. The study involved a group of expectant mothers with a family history of allergies. The mothers were given the probiotic, *L. rhamnosus* GG. The mother's subsequent newborn children were also supplemented with the probiotic for two years. Not only was the prevalence of eczema reduced by half, a four-year follow-up discovered that the preventative effect of the probiotic extended beyond infancy.

Not all of the research has found probiotic supplementation significantly reduces the incidence of atopic dermatitis. A group of researchers studied 178 infants who were considered to be at high risk of allergies because their mothers had allergies. At birth, the infants were randomized to receive either Lactobacillus supplements or a placebo daily for the first six months of life. The infants were assessed for immune function, atopic dermatitis and food allergies at six and 12 months of age. The researchers confirmed that the supplementation was working by checking for Lactobacillius colonization in stool samples; however, no significant differences were found between the groups at either follow-up point. Perhaps certain species are better than others at preventing eczema or there is a particular set or population level of probiotics required. More research is needed, but it appears that probiotics can help reduce eczema and perhaps offer some prevention against its development.

Inflammation and the Intestines: Summary

Probiotics are involved in controlling the inflammation of the intestinal system by promoting defense mechanisms and preventing bad microbes from growing there. Breast-feeding provides probiotics to infants. Infants who have been fed infant formula, and breast-fed infants post-weaning are at risk of invading microbes and can be susceptible to developing inflammation in the intestinal tract. Such inflammation increases the risk of developing allergies.

To date, the research, both in laboratory and clinical settings, suggests that the prevention of atopic eczema in high-risk infants is possible by changing the infant's intestinal microflora with probiotics and prebiotics. Probiotics are effective treatments for atopic dermatitis in infants. Evidence also suggests that probiotics play an important role in controlling immune reactions throughout the body.

Asthma

Problems with the immune system in infancy are not only associated with atopic dermatitis but also with asthma, another atopic disease. Asthma is one of the most common chronic diseases of childhood and the most common causes of school absenteeism. Asthma is inflammation of the bronchial tubes causing airway obstruction, chest tightness, coughing and wheezing.

Asthma commonly develops in people with a history of atopic dermatitis. Studies have shown that school age children with atopic dermatitis (eczema) have an increased risk of developing asthma. This is not surprising as the mucus of the digestive and respiratory systems are very similar. They share many elements involved in immune defense and show some unity in the way they function in an immune response. Clinical investigation has found that people with asthma have an unhealthy microflora in their intestines and tend to have a permeable (leaky) gut. There is a connection between what happens to the mucus that lines the intestines and the lungs. In other words, the intestinal lining and the lungs are connected—a healthy gut can lead to healthy lungs.

Probiotics have been shown to positively affect the atopic disease eczema. Do probiotics have the same positive effect on asthma? Probiotics improve the intestine's ability to fight off invaders through

A healthy gut can lead to healthy lungs. |

What Is Asthma?

Asthma is a chronic disease that affects the airways of the lungs. The inside walls of the airways in a person with asthma are inflamed or swollen. This inflammation makes the airways very sensitive, and they tend to react strongly to allergens. A reaction by the airways to an allergen restricts the movement of air. This causes symptoms such as wheezing, coughing and chest tightness. Asthma cannot be cured, but it can be controlled in most individuals. An asthma attack is a worsening of symptoms in which the muscles around the airways tighten, making the airways narrower and causing less air to flow. An attack can be brought on by an interaction with an allergen or a physiological change in the body. Cells in the airways may also make more mucus than usual. This extra mucus causes further narrowing of the airways. Asthma is an inflammatory-related illness and thus controlling the immune system can help control asthma. The health of the intestinal tract, where 70% of the immune system lies, affects the overall health of the immune system. Unhealthy intestines can worsen asthma symptoms.

their immunological barrier function which reduces the generation of chemicals that promote inflammation and prevents the intestines from becoming permeable. If probiotics are capable of reducing the production of chemicals that promote inflammation involved in allergic reactions, can probiotic supplementation alleviate the symptoms of asthma? Theoretically, this is possible. If probiotics are capable of preventing atopic dermatitis, it is possible that probiotics may also prevent the development of asthma.

Very few clinical studies have found probiotics help fight asthma. *Lactobacillus paracasei-33* is one probiotic species thought to offer benefits to children with asthma. Yet probiotics can play a role in asthma therapy or even prevention. In 2006, scientist Del Giudice and colleagues stated, "In clinical trials probiotics appear to be useful for the treatment of various clinical conditions such as food allergy, atopic dermatitis and allergic rhinitis and in primary prevention of atopy. We can hypothesize that it may be possible, in the future, to use probiotics in primary prevention of asthma."

In 2005, over two million Canadians and about 30 million Americans were suffering from asthma.

Currently, a study is underway in the United States called the Trial of Infant Probiotic Supplementation to Prevent Asthma (TIPS). The TIPS study is based on the hygiene hypothesis, which you have already learned hypothesizes that little or no exposure to bacteria and viruses during a critical period of infancy can lead to problems in the immune system and result in diseases such as asthma. TIPS hopes to determine whether stimulating the immune system with a probiotic supplement, *Lactobacillus rhamnosus* GG, for the first six months of life can prevent or delay asthma development. The three-year study will include about 280 healthy, full-term babies with an increased risk of developing asthma, i.e., either their mother or father has this atopic disease. Studies are also underway in Europe. More will be understood about the potential for probiotics to reduce or treat asthma when the results of these trials are published.

It is not certain whether the ability of probiotics to help with asthma has to do with reducing the chances that the body can become sensitized (allergic to something) or has to do with the ability of probiotics to mature the immune system, which is important in defending against viral infections. There is much more to learn about asthma. With the growing number of children suffering from this disease, we will certainly see more research in this area in the coming years.

Asthma Summary

Probiotics are known to mediate inflammation. This raises the question as to whether probiotic therapy can be used to prevent and treat other inflammatory-based diseases, such as asthma. Population trends suggest that problems with the immune system early in life are linked with an increased risk of developing asthma. Research has suggested that there is a likely connection between probiotics and asthma. Preliminary research confirms that probiotics can improve the quality of life for those with asthma. Ongoing trials hope to give more conclusive answers to how and which probiotics can help treat and perhaps prevent asthma.

FOOD ALLERGIES

A food allergy is an inappropriate immune system response. The body mistakenly believes a food or food particle is harmful. Once the immune system decides a particular food is harmful (labels it as an allergen), it creates specific antibodies to it. As such, the next time the food enters the body, the immune system releases massive amounts of chemicals, including histamine, in an attempt to protect the body from the allergen. These inflammatory chemicals trigger a cascade of allergic symptoms that can affect the skin, intestines, cardiovascular or

Common Sources of Food Allergies
Eggs
Fish
Milk
Peanuts
Shellfish
Soy
Tree Nuts
Wheat

Food Allergy versus Food Intolerance

A food intolerance does not involve the immune system. For example, the food intolerance to lactose, called lactose intolerance, is caused by a lack of the digestive enzyme lactase, which breaks lactose down into its digestible parts. A food allergy occurs when the immune system mistakenly thinks a food particle is foreign and thus elicits an immune or allergic reaction when the food is consumed. This will occur every time this food is consumed; your body has a memory for "foreign" substances.

respiratory system. It has been estimated that approximately 12 million Americans suffer from a food allergy. About 90% of food allergies are caused by soy, shellfish, peanuts, milk, eggs, wheat, tree nuts and fish. The most common action taken to prevent food allergy reactions is to avoid the allergen. However, in a single year, 236 food products were recalled because they contained an allergen not listed on the label or were contaminated with an allergen. Avoidance of a food allergen may not be enough—a means of prevention or treatment is needed.

Food allergies are related to the permeability of the intestinal lining. Inflammation in the intestines causes the lining to become more permeable (leaky), allowing allergens to enter the circulatory system (blood) and cause an allergic reaction. These allergens can include bad microbes and incompletely digested foods.

Normally, the transport of allergens through the intestinal lining to the blood is limited. Thus, a food allergy implies that there is increased leakage between the cells lining the intestinal wall. This is sometimes referred to as **leaky gut syndrome**. This leakage is thought to be caused by a change in the shape of the intestinal cells. This change in shape is caused by toxins that are released by bad microbes living in the intestinal tract. Probiotics are well known to inhibit the presence of bad microbes and reduce the amount of toxins in the intestines. As such, probiotics may prevent leaky gut. Preventing leaky gut can help prevent the uptake of allergens, thus preventing the development of food allergies. Also, by reducing intestinal permeability in those who have food allergies, probiotics may prevent the development of other atopic diseases.

There are three ways in which probiotics are hypothesized to offer beneficial effects in the individuals with food allergies:

1. Children with a food allergy have an increased intestinal permeability. Probiotics have been shown to reverse this, reducing the permeability of the intestines, preventing or treating food allergies.
2. Research has proven that probiotics increase IgA in the intestines. IgA reduces the ability of microbes to adhere to the intestinal lining. This defense is frequently defective in children with food allergies.
3. Changes in number and type of intestinal microbes are common in allergic individuals. Probiotics have the ability to promote a healthy, normal intestinal microflora, thus reducing the development of allergies.

Food Allergies: Summary

Probitics help control the immune reaction to allergies and as such are thought to prevent food allergies. A research study investigated whether probiotics can prevent food allergy development by giving *Bifidobacterium bifidum* and *Lactobacillus casei* to mice with induced allergies. The probiotic decreased the allergic response and appeared to prevent the allergy. Human clinical trials are coming and great excitement lies ahead in the scientific community. If probiotics can in fact prevent or treat food allergies, a great number of people will be helped.

Fatty Inflammation
Dietary lipids, especially long-chain polyunsaturated fatty acids, e.g., omega-3 and omega-6 fatty acids, control immune function. These fats may change the ability of microbes to attach to the intestinal mucus lining. Good fats in the diet are another way to help control immune reactions associated with allergies, and promote a healthy intestine.

Summary

There are more than 400 species of bacteria in the gastrointestinal tract. Only 30 to 40 of these species account for 99% of the microbes that make up the microflora of the human intestinal tract. Some of these species are probiotics. The presence of probiotics in the intestinal tract early in life helps the immune system to mature. Throughout life probiotics reduce the ability of allergens to gain entry into the body and control the immune system to reduce inappropriate reactions known as allergies.

Exposure to allergens early in life can sensitize individuals and lead to the development of allergies. The medical approach to allergic disease is evolving. Instead of trying to avoid allergens, probiotics are being used to prevent the development of allergies by ensuring the immune systems of infants are fully matured and activated. Today, experts believe that the increase in allergic diseases is linked to a lack of stimulation by microbes in the intestines of infants. Probiotics are thought to offer this stimulation. The use of infant formula and increased hygiene practices may be promoting the development of allergies in children by reducing their exposure to probiotics.

A lack of probiotics in the intestinal tract allows bad microbes to grow and release toxins that cause intestinal inflammation. Inflammation in the intestines allows allergens to gain access to the body, leading to sensitization. Probiotics can help reduce the exposure of the body to allergens by reducing the permeability of the intestines. Research suggests that supplementation with probiotics and prebiotics may help the development of a balanced immune defense in infants and children and may reduce the likelihood of developing allergic diseases such as eczema, asthma and food allergies. In clinical practice, probiotics are increasingly being used for these purposes. Probiotics may also help the immune system become strong enough to fight off viral infections, a possible factor in atopic diseases.

chapter
10

Rescue from Lactose Intolerance

A MICROSCOPIC VIEW OF THIS CHAPTER

- Food intolerance is different than a food allergy.
- Lactose intolerance is the inability to digest lactose.
- Probiotics can assist in lactose digestion.
- Lactobacilli contain lactase, which helps break down lactose.
- Bifidobacteria ferment lactose, which helps with its digestion.

■ ■ ■ ■ ■ ■ ■

What is lactose? Lactose is a sugar found in milk and dairy products. In a healthy digestive tract, lactose is broken down into two simpler forms of sugar called glucose and galactose by the enzyme lactase. Glucose and galactose can then be easily absorbed into the blood and used as energy around the body.

Canadian milk consumption has fallen substantially over the past two decades— from about 430 glasses per person in 1980 to 370 glasses in 1999.

Lactose Intolerance versus Milk Intolerance
It is common to confuse lactose intolerance with cow's milk intolerance because the symptoms are often the same. However, the two are not related. Being intolerant to cow's milk is an allergic reaction to proteins in the milk and involves the immune system. Lactose intolerance is a problem with digesting a sugar and thus involves the digestive system.

The majority of the world's population cannot digest lactose. It is estimated that about two-thirds of the world's adult population suffers from lactose maldigestion, also called lactose intolerance. Symptoms include loose stools, abdominal pain, bloating, flatulence and nausea. Typically these symptoms will begin about 30 minutes to two hours after eating or drinking foods containing lactose. The severity of the symptoms will vary depending on the amount of lactose a person can tolerate, a person's age, digestive rate and ethnicity.

Estimated Prevalence of Lactose Intolerance
Native Americans 90%–100%
Asians 90%–100%
Afro-Americans 80%–90%
Mediterranean descendents 80%–90%
Jewish descendents 80%–90%
Northern Europeans 40%–55%

Many humans are unable to properly digest lactose. It is a normal condition in adult mammals and thus cannot be regarded as a disorder. Despite not being classified as a disorder, people who cannot properly digest lactose find this illness causes them a lot of discomfort and requires that they alter their lifestyle and diet. Individuals with lactose intolerance tend to eliminate dairy products from their diet. Dairy products are good sources of dietary calcium and other nutrients. As this illness is not seen as a disorder, these people do not receive proper counseling on how to ensure their diet is rebalanced to ensure they still get sufficient amounts of calcium and other key nutrients. Lactose intolerance is a major health problem. It can result in dietary deficiencies in nutrients, such as calcium, and this can lead to degenerative diseases including osteoporosis.

Two major types of lactose maldigestion can occur. At birth, the enzyme β-galactosidase, more commonly known as lactase, is present in high quantities. Yet, as we become children and adolescents, the concentration of lactase in our digestive system decreases and we are less able to digest lactose.

> **Non-Dairy Dietary Sources of Calcium**
> Dairy is not the only source of calcium, despite misleading representations on North American Food Guides. Millions of Asians who use the Chinese food guide, called The Pagoda, are told about dairy equivalents. Appendix 12-1 has a more complete list of calcium food sources. These include:
> broccoli
> bok choy
> kale
> sardines
> salmon
> almonds
> sesame seeds

The second type of lactose maldigestion is caused by a loss of mucus on the lining of the small intestine. This happens in cases of diarrhea or bowel resection. A loss in intestinal mucosa is a problem for lactose digestion. Lactase is produced by the cells that line the small intestine. The loss of intestinal mucosa is an unhealthy event for these cells. Less lactase is produced, in turn, reducing the ability of the body to properly digest lactose. As such, it is no surprise that lactose maldigestion is frequently experienced by adults who suffer from acute or chronic enteritis or bowel resection.

Certain probiotic species are capable of helping with lactose digestion. Lactobacilli species can help digest lactose. Lactobacilli can produce the enzyme lactase. Bifidobacteria use fermentation to break down lactose. As such, those suffering from lactose intolerance may benefit from consuming a variety of probiotic species.

LACTOBACILLI FOR LACTOSE INTOLERANCE

One of the first beneficial effects of probiotics ever demonstrated was their ability to ease lactose intolerance. Perhaps it started with the observation that lactose-intolerant individuals can handle the lactose in yogurt better than that found in milk. This is likely because yogurt is also a source of lactase, the enzyme that aids in the breakdown of lactose in the digestive system. When the bacteria (Lactobacilli) in the yogurt are broken open by the bile salts in the small intestine, they release high levels of lactase in the gastrointestinal tract. Lactase acts on the lactose and aids in its proper digestion. When there is no undigested lactose in the intestinal track, there is no discomfort, and other lactose intolerant symptoms.

Lactose-intolerant adults tolerate yogurt better than milk.

Clinical trials have tried to identify which probiotic species offer the best reduction in lactose intolerance symptoms. One of the most common bacteria species found in yogurt is *Lactobacillus acidophilus*. *L. acidophilus* is a lactase-containing bacteria. However, *L. acidophilus* has a higher resistance to bile and thus it may not break down as well as other bacteria. This may explain why preliminiary clinical trials in which *L. acidophilus* was given in supplement form do not show significant improvements in lactose intolerance symptoms.

The study was conducted just before 2000. Subjects took the strain *Lactobacillus acidophilus* BG2FO4 twice daily for seven days in a randomized, controlled human trial. The results were not statistically significant and failed to produce convincing evidence that this species eliminated lactose intolerance in these subjects.

A study using milk containing *L. acidophilus* and *L. bulgaricus* confirmed that *L. acidophilus* is not the best choice for lactose-intolerant people. They both have similar abilities to produce lactase, but *L. bulgaricus* is superior for those with lactose intolerance. It has a cell structure that allows its lactase to more easily enter the intestines. In fact, *L. bulgaricus* was found in the study to effectively assist with lactose digestion in those who suffered from lactose intolerance.

It is likely that other probiotic supplements can help improve lactose intolerance symptoms. VSL#3 is a blend of probiotics produced by Seaford Pharmaceuticals in Ontario, Canada. It has been used in a number of clinical trials. Some studies noted in other chapters of this book have found this supplement has positive results on health; however, VSL#3 does not appear to assist in lactose intolerance. In a clinical study, VSL#3 was given to 10 volunteers for one or four days. Two weeks later, a lactose challenge was carried out by the volunteers. No statistically significant changes were observed, but there was a trend toward improvement. To date, the research does not suggest that this combination of probiotics is effective in treating lactose intolerance.

Current research is working to discover probiotic strains, which are rapidly destroyed by bile in the small intestine. These strains can be carriers of lactase into the body to help with lactose digestion. These probiotics will help with lactose digestion and potentially will alleviate lactose intolerance more efficiently. For now, having a healthy Lactobacilli population in the small intestine and consuming yogurt over other dairy products are strategies that can be used by people who suffer from lactose intolerance.

Some experts suggest that it is not the Lactobacilli that are so important, but Bifidobacteria that improve lactose intolerance symptoms.

BIFIDOBACTERIA FOR LACTOSE INTOLERANCE

Lactose intolerance can be reduced by lactase released into the small intestine when Lactobacilli are broken down by bile salts. Probiotics may also play a helpful role in lactose intolerance in the large intestine. When researchers compared the differences in lactose intolerance symptoms in volunteers, they found that their symptoms were caused by differences in the colon's ability to break down lactose. In other words, it may not be the lactase from probiotics in the small intestine that aids symptoms of lactose intolerance, but the fermentation of lactose by probiotics in the colon. As such, changing the probiotic colonies in the colon may help lactose digestion. The probiotics best suited to do this are Bifidobacteria, the most prominent probiotics in the colon.

Bifidobacterium longum has been investigated as a potential probiotic treatment for lactose intolerance. It appears to have a positive effect. In a study, 11 lactose-intolerant volunteers were given a capsule (*B. longum*) and yogurt (*B. animalis, L. bulgaricus* and *S. thermophilus*) respectively for 14 days. The subjects were given a food containing lactose to see how these probiotics helped them digest it. The researchers found that taking the high dosages of Bifidobacteria was helpful. The probiotics made it through the stomach and small intestine and were living in the colon. The Bifidobacteria in the yogurt and supplement caused an increase in the number of Bifidobacteria living in the colon of the 11 volunteers. Bifidobacteria are effective fermentors of lactose and other carbohydrates. The volunteers noted improvements in their ability to handle lactose-containing foods. Bifidobacteria appear to play an important role in alleviating lactose intolerance symptoms.

SUMMARY

Clinical research on probiotics and lactose intolerance suggests that an increased number of probiotics in the intestinal tract might contribute to the reduction of lactose intolerance symptoms. It is thought that the release of lactase by broken Lactobacilli in the small intestine and fermentation of lactose by Bifidobacteria in the colon help reduce the symptoms of lactose intolerance. The use of both families of probiotics may be helpful for people with lactose intolerance. Probiotic strains behave differently, and there is some evidence that suggests certain strains, concentrations and preparations are likely effective against lactose intolerance. Which strain or concentration is best is yet to be discovered.

chapter
11

The Urogenital Tract and Probiotics: Yeast Buster and More

A Microscopic View of This Chapter

- Microbes also live in the urogenital tract.
- Probiotics support health in the urogenital tract.
- Use of probiotics can help fight yeast overgrowth.
- Vaginal bacteriosis is caused by overgrowth of bad microbes.
- Probiotics may help prevent and treat urinary tract infections.
- Oral and intravaginal administration of probiotics supports the urogenital tract.

■ ■ ■ ■ ■ ■ ■

The microflora that exists in our body does not just live in the gastrointestinal tract. Microbes can move from place to place, and the microflora in our body will move from the mouth, throughout the intestinal tract and into the urogenital (urethra and bladder) tract. Some microbes also live on your skin. The microflora needs no passport. There are no borders between these areas of the body. The movement of microbes is unrestricted. Of note, their movement does not happen at great lengths, as each species has a preferred location to live in the body. An example is Bifidobacteria's preference to colonize in the large intestine.

You can find microbes in the mouth, intestinal tract, urethra, vagina and on the skin. The urogenital tract consists of the urethra and bladder (and vagina in females). The urogenital tract is normally sterile with the exception of the vagina and the distal first centimeter of the urethra. This small population of microbes in the urogenital tract may not compare to the large numbers found in the intestines, but its influence on the body's health is almost as important.

How do Lactobacilli promote a healthy urogenital tract? These organisms lower the pH of the vagina to 4 or 5, which inhibits the growth of bad microbes. If conditions change, such as an increase in stress or the use of antibiotics, the presence of Lactobacilli declines. If there is a loss in the number of Lactobacilli in the urogenital tract, the defenses available to fight bad microbes are decreased. Where do these bad microbes come from? The origin of the bad microbes in urinary tract infections and bacterial vaginosis commonly comes from fecal flora.

Bad microbes that can thrive in a urogenital tract that lacks Lactobacilli include *Candida albicans*, Streptococci and *E. coli*. When conditions are favorable toward these bad microbes, they flourish, causing disease or illness in the urogential tract. Such diseases include Candida infections (yeast infection), bacteria vaginosis and urinary tract infections. Urogenital infections are a problem shared worldwide. They are the most common reason for a woman to decide to visit a gynecologist or urologist.

Research has discovered that the presence of certain probiotics appears to lessen the severity of some of these urogenital illnesses. Lactobacilli are thought to play a major role in the health of the urogenital tract.

THE VAGINA

The vagina, also called the birth canal, is a thin-walled tube about 8 to 10 centimeters long. It lies between the bladder and rectum. It extends from the cervix, the opening to the uterus, to the outside of the body. The vagina provides a passageway for the delivery of an infant and for menstrual flow to leave the body. As the vagina is a passageway between the outside environment and the body, it is a common place to find microbes. In close proximity to the anus, the vagina can easily be infected with bacteria from the large intestine. Bad microbes from feces can easily find their way over to the vagina.

Various members of the Lactobacillus family love to live in the vagina. Certain Bifidobacteria also live in the vagina, although everyone is different. We have different genes, different fingerprints and different microflora. There is no one dominant probiotic species in a healthy vagina. The dominant species of bacteria in one woman's vagina may be different than the next. However, we do know that Lactobacilli are common in all healthy vaginas, and they have a protective effect against the colonization and overgrowth of bad microbes.

Some studies have tried to identify which species are commonly found in healthy vaginal microflora. Both Bifidobacteria and Lactobacilli species are present. Four species—*Bifidobacterium bifidum, B. breve, B. adolescentis* and *B. longum*—are thought to be the dominant Bifidobacteria in the vaginal microflora. Little research has been done in the area of Bifidobacteria and the vagina, but as these species are also common in the large intestine, it is not surprising that they are found inhabiting the vagina as well.

Lactobacilli have long been considered the protective microbes of the vagina. An investigation of 19 healthy women discovered that *Lactobacillus gasseri* was the dominant Lactobacilli in their vaginas. However, there is no consensus among experts that this species is the most important or universally dominant vaginal probiotic. *Lactobacillus crispatus, Lactobacillus jensenii* and *Lactobacillus vaginalis* have also been identified as important species in the vagina. Natural differences from human to human likely explain the conflicting results as to which probiotic species is the most dominant in the vagina.

With no consensus on which Lactobacilli are most dominant, a group of scientists sought to discover which species of Lactobacilli were most effective. *Lactobacillus acidophillus* CRL 1259 and *Lactobacillus paracasei* CRL 1289 were found to inhibit bad microbes, such as *Staphylococcus aureus*, from attaching to the lining of the vagina. More strains are likely to be found to offer similar protective effects against vaginal infections. Lactobacilli play an important role in maintaining urogential health.

How does oral supplementation of probiotics affect the vagina? The vagina is not part of the gastrointestinal tract. Probiotics move from the rectum to the vagina and/or cause changes in the body that promote probiotic growth in the vagina. Oral probiotic supplementation positively changes the diversity of microbes in the vagina. Probiotics are also available as suppositories, which work very well; however, research does not support this method as a superior administration route to oral supplementation.

Yeast Infections

In a healthy vagina, probiotics are dominant. They are present in large, healthy colonies. They stimulate the immune system and create an environment that inhibits the growth of bad microbes. However, there are many conditions that can tip the balance: stress, antibiotic use, consuming foods that contain antibiotics, environmental changes and infection. By altering the balance of microflora in the vagina, bad microbes can flourish. The result is an infection, inflammation or other illness. Candida overgrowth and bacteria vaginosis are both examples of illnesses that can arise when the delicate balance of microbes in the vagina is altered and bad microbes flourish.

It is estimated that 70% of the female population has suffered from Candida-related symptoms at some point in their lives. An overgrowth of Candida is called *Candidiasis*. Candida is a yeast that lives in us and on us as part of our body's normal collection of microbes. In a normal digestive tract, about 90% of the body's Candida live in the mouth and colon. *Candida albicans* is most often the species of Candida found on the skin and in the vagina of humans. The stomach, small and large intestine are hostile to Candida growth, so not much is found there. As such, Candida overgrowth is commonly only seen on the skin or in the vagina.

A Candida infection is also called a yeast infection.

A yeast infection is a horrible experience. Symptoms of a yeast infection include itching, burning, redness and irritation of the vaginal area. Severe yeast infections may cause swelling of the vulva. In some cases women experience painful and/or frequent urination, which is caused by inflammation of the urinary opening. Excessive vaginal discharge, which is thicker than normal, appears whiter, curd-like and looks

About 70% of females have experienced a yeast overgrowth.

similar to cottage cheese, will be apparent in women experiencing vaginal yeast infections.

The vagina may increase mucus production and encourage candida overgrowth as a reaction to contact al-

Conditions that promote yeast overgrowth: environmental changes, stress, using antibiotics, bacterial infection and eating allergenic foods.

lergens and circulating food allergens. For example, a milk allergy commonly triggers inflammation and Candida overgrowth in both children and adults. Yeast overgrowth can be a nuisance. There is no way to eliminate all of the yeast in your body. All you can hope is to find a balance in which yeast grows at a controlled rate below levels that cause symptoms. Probiotics can help you find this balance.

Yeast in Men?

Yeast overgrowth is not isolated in women. Men can suffer symptoms of yeast overgrowth. It is more common than you may think. Men may be troubled by yeast overgrowth on their penis or on the skin around the anus and groin. This is more commonly known as "jock itch." Sexual intercourse can transfer yeast from a man to a woman. Both partners should consider probiotic treatment.

Antibiotic use changes the bacteria in the vagina and thus promotes the growth of Candida. Antibiotic use reduces the presence of all bacteria, including the beneficial probiotics in the vagina such as Lactobacillus. Antibiotic use causes the vaginal probiotic population to shrink. Then the pH of the vagina increases, due to no lactic acid coming from Lactobacilli to keep it low, and Candida is no longer restricted. Candida can colonize and flourish in such an environment.

How do Lactobacilli inhibit and control Candida? According to laboratory studies, Lactobacilli reduces the ability of *Candida albicans* to attach to the cells that line the vagina (vaginal epithelium), thus restricting its ability to colonize in the vagina.

The birth control pill also alters the vaginal environment. Many women use the birth control pill. It inhibits ovulation by altering hormone levels in the body. The use of birth control pills has been strongly linked to the development of *Candidiasis*. The birth control pill can disrupt the delicate balance of bacteria in the body, and allow yeast to grow. Probiotics have the ability to prevent yeast's ability to grow. As such, probiotics offer women, particularly those on birth control pills or using antibiotics, a defense against Candida.

Many species of probiotics are known to inhibit *Candida albicans* growth in the vagina. In particular, *Lactobacillus acidophilus*, *Lactobacillus rhamnosus* GR-1 and *Lactobacillus fermentum* RC-14 taken orally or intravaginally are strains that can effectively fight against Candida. The use of Lactobacilli species to combat Candida is a good choice for women. More research is still needed in this area. In the meantime, the use of probiotics should be considered by women with frequent recurrences of Candida infections, as probiotics offer many immune health benefits—and adverse reactions from probiotics are very rare, unlike commonly prescribed antifungal agents.

Bacterial Vaginosis

Bacterial vaginosis is a condition in which the number of Lactobacilli in the vagina decrease and an overgrowth of bad microbes occurs. Bacterial vaginosis has been associated with various gynecological and obstetric complications as discussed in Chapter 7.

Bacterial vaginosis is commonly treated with antibiotics. As such, it has an extremely high recurrence rate. This may be because antibiotics do not help the underlying problem of bacterial vaginosis—an imbalance of microbes in the vagina. Antibiotics do not just kill bad bacteria, including *Gardnerella vaginalis*, a common cause of bacterial vaginosis; they also kill all of the bacteria in the body, including probiotics. The result is similar to an empty parking lot. After antibiotic use, the lot is empty and it is a race between all microbes to grab a parking spot. By repopulating the parking lot with probiotics as soon as possible, there are fewer spots open for pathogenic microbes. Antibiotic treatment of bacterial vaginosis does not help establish healthy microbes in the vagina. Consuming probiotics during and after antibiotic use decreases the risk of bad microbes growing in the body and causing disease. The use of high-potency

> *By repopulating the parking lot with probiotics as soon as possible, there are fewer spots for bad microbes.*

probiotics during and after antibiotic use offers the most beneficial effects. Women with bacterial vaginosis using antibiotic therapy can benefit from probiotic use.

Scientists have been studying the characteristics of probiotic strains that naturally live in a healthy urogential tract. Probiotics that are effective in preventing bacterial infections have the following characteristics:

- They prevent the growth of bad microbes.
- They can produce acid and hydrogen peroxide.
- They can attach to the cells of the vagina (vaginal epithelial cells).
- Strains thought to offer these characteristics include: *L. acidophilus* 61701 and *L. acidophilus* 48101, as well as *L. crispatus* 55730 and *L. delbrueckii* 65407. *Lactobacillus rhamnosus* is thought to offer the best potential against bacterial vaginosis. Lactobacilli are particularly effective at preventing bacterial vaginosis.

In a human clinical trial, 10 billion (10^{10}) colony-forming units of *L. rhamnosus* were given orally to 10 women daily for two weeks. The women were suffering from abnormal flora in their vagina. The majority of the women complained of pains, frequent urination and vaginal irritation prior to the study. Within one week of probiotic introduction into their daily routine, the women reported a disappearance of their symptoms. Most exciting was the follow-up reports from the women; they had a healthy vaginal flora for several months following supplementation. Probiotics can help you rebalance your vaginal flora and the effects last for a few months. This is great news for women who suffer from recurrent vaginal infections.

Combinations of probiotics are also effective. *Lactobacillus rhamnosus* in combination with *Lactobacillus fermentum* has positive effects on the vaginal tract. In a study of 42 females with bacterial vaginosis, a daily oral dose of one billion (10^9) colony-forming units of *L. rhamnosus* and *L. fermentum* for one month treated 70% of the cases. There were no reported side effects in this study. The researchers also tested *L. rhamnosus* GG in this trial, but it did not have any effect on the bacterial vaginosis.

What is the best probiotic combination to fight bacterial vaginosis? To date, there are no conclusions as to the perfect mix of probiotic strains to cure bacterial vaginosis; however, it appears that Lactobacilli offers the best effects and is a potential treatment. The evidence strongly associates a healthy vaginal microflora with a reduced risk of developing bacterial vaginosis. Probiotics may be a good way to prevent bacterial vaginosis.

PREBIOTICS FOR VAGINAL HEALTH

Prebiotics beneficially affect you by stimulating the growth and activity of probiotics. As such, prebiotics may help increase the probiotic populations in the vagina and help prevent or treat yeast infections or bacterial vaginosis.

Specific research has investigated whether prebiotics selectively promote the growth of probiotics in the vaginal tract without promoting the growth of bad microbes in the vagina. Of 17 Lactobacilli strains found in healthy vaginas, three that were deemed dominant were selected for a prebiotic study. Four prebiotics were tested, including two fructooligosaccharides (FOS) and two glucooligosaccharides (GOS). Two of the prebiotics (FOS Actilight DP3 and alpha-1,4 GOS DP) were only used by the Lactobacilli strains. Common bad microbes in the vagina were unable to metabolize these prebiotics. Therefore, prebiotics do help good microbes grow and do not stimulate the growth of bad microbes. Prebiotics are a way to help the vagina stay healthy.

URINARY TRACT INFECTIONS

Traditionally, probiotics are used to improve gastrointestinal health; however, the urogenital tract also has microbes, and disturbance of this microflora may lead to urinary tract infections.

Infections of the urinary tract are the second most common type of infection in the body. Women are especially prone to urinary tract infections for reasons that are not yet well understood. One woman in five develops a urinary tract infection during her lifetime. In men, urinary tract infections are not as common as in women, but they can be very serious when they do occur.

How does a urinary tract infection occur? Normally, urine is sterile (free of bacteria,

viruses and fungi). An infection occurs when microorganisms, usually bacteria from the digestive tract, cling to the opening of the urethra and begin to multiply. The urethra is the tube that carries urine from the bladder to outside the body. An infection limited to the urethra is called urethritis. However, bacteria can move up the urethra and infect the bladder. A bladder infection is called cystitis. This type of infection is of concern, for if it is not treated promptly, the bacteria colonizing in the bladder can move up the ureters into the kidneys and result in a kidney infection. A kidney infection is called *pyelonephritis*.

Microorganisms that commonly cause a urinary tract infection include *Chlamydia*, *Mycoplasma*, *Gardnerella vaginalis* and most frequently *E. coli*. Unlike *E. coli*, whose source tends to be feces, *Chlamydia* and *Mycoplasma* are sexually transmitted, and these infections require treatment of both partners.

Luckily, the urinary system is structured in a way that helps ward off infections by bacteria. The natural downward flow of urine makes it hard for bacterial to move up the tract. Urine indirectly washes bacteria in the urinary tract out of the body. Also, the ureters and bladder normally

---

The Urinary Tract

The urinary tract is made up of the kidneys, ureters, urinary bladder and the urethra. The kidneys filter the blood and continually make urine, which is carried by the ureters to the bladder, where it is stored until it is convenient to release it. The average adult passes about a quart and a half of urine each day and the volume formed at night is about half that formed in the daytime. The urethra is a thin-walled tube that carries urine by peristalsis from the bladder to the outside of the body. The length and relative function of the urethra differs among men and women. In females, the urethra is about three to four centimeters long and its external end is in front of the vaginal opening. In males, the urethra is about 20 centimeters long and not only carries urine but also carries sperm.

prevent urine from backing up toward the kidneys. In men, the prostate gland produces secretions that slow bacterial growth. In both sexes, immune defenses along the lining of the urinary tract prevent infection. Probiotics increase these immune defenses and guard the lining of the urinary tract. Probiotics help reduce the risk of infection.

There is a high incidence of urogenital infections of bacterial origin among the world's female population during their reproductive years.

Recurrent urinary tract infections bother a great number of women around the world. Although this area has been rarely investigated, probiotics that produce hydrogen peroxide appear to reduce the risk of urinary tract infections. In particular, the use of Lactobacilli has been considered for the prevention of urinary tract infections. Lactobacilli are the dominant species in the urogenital tract of healthy premenopausal women. As such, supplementing with Lactobacilli probiotics may protect against urinary tract infections.

Many studies (in vitro, animal experiments, microbiological studies, clinical trials) have looked at the ability of probiotics to help fight bad microbes that cause urinary tract infections. Most of the studies have produced encouraging findings. *Lactobacillus rhamnosus* and *L. reuteri* seem to be the most effective at preventing urinary tract infections among the studied species of Lactobacilli. Most studies used oral supplementation; however, vaginal insertion may also offer positive effects. A study noted that vaginal insertion of probiotic suppositories containing *L. rhamnosus* or *L. fermentum* decreased the rates of urinary tract infection by up to 75% with no adverse effects reported. Other probiotics, including *L. casei* Shirota and *L. crispatus* have also shown efficacy in some studies. *L. rhamnosus* GG did not appear to be quite as effective. The evidence from the available studies suggests that probiotics can prevent recurrent urinary tract infections in women.

L. rhamnosus, L. reuteri and *L. fermentum, L. casei* Shirota and *L. crispatus* are good species to consider when choosing a probiotic to fight urogential infections. Of note, other Lactobacilli species are probably effective in fighting urogenital infections as they boost immunity and inhibit the growth of bad microbes throughout the body.

SUMMARY

Just as the microflora of the intestinal tract plays a role in health, the microflora of the urogenital tract also plays an important role in health. Preliminary research in this area suggests that probiotics are vital in maintaining a healthy urogenital tract. Growth of bad microbes can result in Candida infections, urinary tract infections and bacterial vaginosis. Keeping a healthy population of probiotics in the urogenital tract can help prevent these illnesses. Supplementation both orally and vaginally shows promise as treatments for infections of the urogential tract caused by bad microbe overgrowth. Probiotics present in the rectum are capable of translocating to the urogenital tract to elicit beneficial effects. The research in this area is still young in its development. How probiotics cause their positive effects is not known for certain; however, the mechanisms are likely to be similar to those seen in the intestinal tract. Some species have been shown to offer specific benefits to the host. Lactobacilli are likely to emerge as an effective species for vaginal health. Future research is required to determine which probiotic species combinations are most effective against urogenital infections.

chapter
12

Probiotics for Strong Bones

A Microscopic View of This Chapter

- Bones are continually breaking down and rebuilding.
- Nutrients, like calcium, are required to keep bones healthy.
- Calcium in bones is used in muscle contractions and to balance blood pH.
- Probiotics promote proper digestion and absorption of nutrients.
- Vitamin K2, created by probiotics, supports bone growth.
- Prebiotics increase the absorption of bone-building nutrients.

■ ■ ■ ■ ■ ■ ■

Bones are the hardest part of your body. They are the scaffolding our muscles and organs cling too. Without bones we would be globs of tissue without the ability to run and jump. We all understand the great importance of our bones. As we age, the loss of bone integrity (low bone mass) can be debilitating, restricting our quality of life. Broken hips and backs leave many older adults reliant on wheelchairs and limited in their ability to move and function. Be good to your bones to ensure they are strong and stable for many years to come. Let's be sure our healthy bones will support us in activities like playing golf and gardening when we retire.

HEALTHY DIGESTION FOR HEALTHY BONES

Ensuring your bones are healthy requires the digestion and absorption of nutrients. First, you need to make sure your diet is rich in calcium, phosphorus, magnesium, vitamin D and vitamin K. Vegetables, nuts and dairy foods are great sources of these nutrients.

By 2020, 62 million North Americans are expected to suffer from low bone mass.

Bone-building nutrients cannot get to their destination if they are not properly digested and absorbed. Your enzymes control the pathways of digestion and absorption. Enzymes are proteins that your body makes every day to help you function. To ensure these enzymes are present in high enough amounts requires that you eat the right foods. Since enzymes are proteins, they are built using amino acids. A diet rich in amino acids (found in beans, corn, meats, nuts, seeds) ensures you have the nutrients needed to build these enzymes. There is yet another important factor involved in your ability to get bone-building nutrients to your bones—probiotics. Probiotics influence the absorption of nutrients involved in bone health.

About 70% of North American adults suffer from maldigestion, malabsorption, digestive illnesses and unhealthy bacteria in the digestive tract.

PROBIOTICS FOR BONE HEALTH

Probiotics have a powerful impact on your digestive system. When undesirable and unhealthy microbes such as yeast, fungus and bad bacteria start to proliferate in the gastrointestinal tract, they quickly change the intestines, triggering inflammation, which cascades into a reduced ability to digest and absorb nutrients needed for healthy bones.

Improper absorption in the intestinal tract can lead to a lack of essential nutrients required by the bones and other parts of the body. Not being able to properly absorb food reduces the amount of bone-building nutrients available to the bones. A lack of nutrients to the bones can lead to significant bone loss, according to researchers. Therefore, maintaining a healthy flora in the intestinal tract helps make sure you are absorbing the most nutrients possible. Probiotics ensure that the nutrients you swallow make their way to the bones that need them. Probiotics appear to play an important role in bone health.

Despite the common misconception that bones are hard, lifeless parts of the human body, bones are actually active tissue. Bone cells are constantly breaking down and rebuilding. Why do bones break down? Bone is broken down to offer the body minerals it needs to maintain homeostasis. Your bones are your body's reservoir of calcium. Every muscle contraction you do requires a calcium ion. That's right. Every time you blink, you use calcium. All day long, you are using calcium and requiring your bones to break down.

Calcium is also used to help maintain the pH of your blood. When your blood pH levels drop, or becomes more acidic, your body uses some of the calcium stored in the bones to rebalance the blood pH. Eating certain foods (processed foods, soda pop) can cause an acidic shift in your blood. This is the basis for some raw food diets which try to focus on eating foods that do not cause an acidic shift in your blood pH, thus keeping your calcium levels healthy all day long. If you continually use calcium from your bones, you will lose some of your bone mineral density, causing your bones to become weak. Eating healthy foods that help ensure your blood levels of calcium are good is important to bone health. Fruits and vegetables do not pull calcium from your bones. Eat these healthy foods more often and your bones will thank you.

Including sources of calcium in your diet throughout the day can help ensure there is available calcium to help balance your blood pH and help your muscles contract; ultimately, this reduces your need to pull calcium from your bones. What types of foods can you include in your daily diet that provide calcium? Try raisins on your cereal in the morning, eat low-fat yogurt or cheese in your lunch or as mid-day snacks, include green leafy vegetables or fish in your dinner. Appendix 12-1 lists food items that contain calcium.

How Much Calcium Do You Need?

According to the United States Dietary Association, children (one to eight years old) need 500–800 mg per day, teenagers (nine to 18 years old) need 1,300 mg per day, adult men and women need 1,000 mg per day and people over the age of 50 need 1,200 mg per day. A list of other food sources of calcium is listed in Appendix 12-1.

WHAT OTHER NUTRIENTS DO YOUR BONES NEED?

Calcium cannot do its critical work alone. Calcium needs an entire team of bone-building nutrients to keep your bones healthy and strong. Other nutrients in the bone-building team include: vitamin B6, vitamin B9, vitamin B12, vitamin D3, vitamin C, and trace minerals boron, magnesium, calcium, silicon, copper and zinc. Another essential bone-building nutrient is vitamin K2, a nutrient that is not easy to serve up on your plate.

Osteoporosis is estimated to affect about 75 million people in Europe, the USA and Japan.

Vitamin K and Bone Health

There are two types of vitamin K involved in your bone health. Vitamin K1, or *phylloquinone*, is found in any green vegetables such as lettuce, broccoli and spinach, and makes up about 90% of the vitamin K found in a typical Western diet. Vitamin K2 is the more biologically active form and is called *menaquinones*. Certain probiotics are capable of converting vitamin K1 into vitamin K2. Probiotics convert vitamin K1 in the intestines into vitamin K2. Vitamin K2 is found in egg yolk, butter and fermented soy foods; it makes up about 10% of the vitamin K consumed in a typical Western diet.

Why do you need vitamin K2? Vitamin K2 helps the body turn on biological switches that activate three critical proteins: osteocalcin, calcitonin and matrix G1a. Osteocalcin, calcitonin and matrix G1a are calcium-binding proteins that are essential in guiding calcium into the bone. In particular, these proteins ensure calcium reaches the osteoblast cells of the bone, which are the cells responsible for making bone. Not having enough vitamin K2 in your body can cause calcium to deposit in soft tissues such as the arteries, heart and brain because there are not enough proteins directing calcium correctly to the bones. Calcium deposition in the arteries of the heart and brain can promote plaque formation and clots leading to heart attacks or strokes. Interestingly, the *Journal of the American College of Cardiology* in 2000 stated that having too low a level of vitamin K2 raised the risk of heart attacks by 2.4 times. We need vitamin K2 to help our bones and reduce our risk of heart attacks. Since probiotics help us create vitamin K2, one could say that we need probiotics for our bones and our hearts.

Researchers have confirmed in studies that vitamin K2 plays a significant role in bone health. A double-blind,

Probiotics enhance the conversion of vitamin K1, the predominant form of vitamin K in the diet, into the bone-healthy vitamin K2.

placebo-controlled study, by researchers at Maastricht University and the Cardiovascular Research Institute, followed 325 healthy women with no osteoporosis for three years. The researchers found that vitamin K2 supplements boosted the women's bone mineral content, compared to placebo. A Harvard Medical School study confirmed the efficacy of vitamin K2 to prevent bone loss and noted that it reduces the rate of vertebral fractures. Other studies also suggest vitamin K2 plays a role in bone health.

Ensuring sufficient vitamin K2 is available in your body appears to be important to ensuring not just bone health, but also reducing the risk of heart attacks and strokes. Probiotics enhance the conversion of vitamin K1, the predominant form of vitamin K in the diet, into the bone healthy vitamin K2. Keeping your intestinal probiotic population at high levels throughout your life may help reduce the risk of bone loss and other diseases. Yogurt, supplements and prebiotics can help keep your probiotic colonies happy and healthy.

PREBIOTICS

Prebiotics can help support the health of probiotics in your intestines. This may help increase the ability of your digestive tract to absorb bone-building nutrients and convert vitamin K1 into vitamin K2.

Several studies in animals and humans have shown prebiotics have positive effects on mineral absorption and metabolism as well as on bone composition and architecture. Prebiotics including inulin, oligofructose, fructooligosaccharides and galactooligosaccharides are great additions to a bone-healthy diet. The ability of prebiotics to improve your bone health depends on your chronological age, physiological age, menopausal status and your ability to absorb calcium.

There are many underlying mechanisms by which prebiotics enhance mineral absorption. On the following page is a list of the mechanisms by which prebiotics can improve mineral absorption and bone health.

All in all, the end result is a healthier environment in the intestines in which more minerals and vitamins can be absorbed. Prebiotics:

- stabilize the intestinal flora and ecology
- improve gut health, thus improving absorption and digestion
- increase the release of bone-modulating factors from foods, e.g., phytoestrogens
- enhance probiotic activity, including production of short-chain fatty acids, which increase the solubility of minerals
- promote probiotic health by enhancing metabolism of vitamin K1 into vitamin K2 and thus increasing the expression of calcium-binding proteins
- promote health of microflora which produces fermentation products that promote proliferation of intestinal cells, called *enterocytes*, which ultimately increase absorption surface area and increase nutrient uptake.

In short, prebiotics can help promote healthy bones. Many research studies have shown prebiotics to have the ability to improve factors that promote bone health. One study found that bone mineral density was improved in rats who were given a prebiotic supplement. In fact, the researchers reported that the fructooligosaccharides, the prebiotic, reversed the loss of bone thickness and separation. Prebiotics lead to healthy bones.

Prebiotics stimulate the absorption of nutrients in the intestinal tract and improve bone mineralization. A lot of the evidence supporting the use of prebiotics to improve bone health comes from animal experiments. In the studies, prebiotics increase the availability of calcium, magnesium, zinc, and iron, all of which are minerals needed for healthy bones. Human trials have confirmed that prebiotics improve your body's ability to absorb bone-building nutrients. Since prebiotics are best known for their ability to support the growth of probiotics, we may associate the bone-healthy effects of prebiotics with probiotics. However, studies suggest that the effects of prebiotics are different than those of probiotics in terms of bone health.

You've seen that prebiotics are healthy for your bones, so how do you get them into your diet? Prebiotics are the indigestible fiber found in many foods. Prebiotics are present in raw fruits, vegetables and grains and nuts. Manufacturers of foods are adding prebiotics to packaged foods. As fiber, prebiotics are perfect ingredients to add to packaged foods as they do not affect taste, moisture or shelf-life of the product. One of the most common group of prebiotics added to packaged foods is called *fructooligosaccharides*, declared as FOS, (a short form of fructooligosaccharide) on the label. You may also see it called *NutraFlora*, a popular brand found in North American products. Added to yogurt, cereal and many other foods, prebiotics offer a shelf-stable, tasteless, convenient way to promote better nutrient absorption and stronger bones.

SUMMARY

A healthy microflora supports the health and function of the gastrointestinal tract. Probiotics promote proper nutrient digestion and absorption. Nutrient absorption provides bones with the team of nutrients required to keep this active tissue healthy. The bones are a reserve for calcium used to support muscle contractions and stabilize changes in the blood pH. Calcium absorption is vital to the health of your bones and your overall health.

Calcium is guided into the bones by vitamin K2. This vitamin is not commonly found in your diet. Probiotics can convert vitamin K1 to vitamin K2, which helps to successfully guide calcium into your 206 bones, promoting strong bone growth and likely helping to reduce the risk of developing osteoporosis. Vitamin K2 boosts the formation of healthy bones, helps maintain healthy bones, slows and may even stop bone loss and plays a role in blood clotting. Without vitamin K2, calcium can deposit in your arteries, increasing the risk of heart attack and stroke. The effects of probiotics reach beyond the confinements of the intestinal tract and can elicit a positive effect on bone health. Probiotics promote a healthy body with strong bones.

Prebiotics have a number of beneficial effects on the microflora in your intestine, and they promote the absorption of bone-building nutrients. Prebiotic supplementation appears to enhance bone health in both animal and human studies. Consuming foods that naturally contain prebiotics or those with added prebiotics, such as fructoligosaccharides, may be a bone-healthy choice.

chapter
13

Heart Attack: Probiotics and Their Effect on Cholesterol

A MICROSCOPIC VIEW OF THIS CHAPTER

- Cholesterol is a contributing factor to heart disease.
- High serum cholesterol levels contribute to atherosclerosis.
- Atherosclerosis hardens the arteries and leads to heart attacks and strokes.
- Probiotics lower cholesterol levels.
- Bile salt hydrolase in probiotics reduces the cholesterol reabsorption in the gut.
- Bifidobacteria contain bile salt hydrolase as do some Lactobacilli species.
- Probiotics may help your heart by lowering blood pressure.

■ ■ ■ ■ ■ ■ ■

Heart disease is the number one killer in Western society. There are many factors that contribute to heart disease including stress, lack of exercise, diet and cholesterol. In fact, there are over 286 risk factors for heart disease. Gender, age and weight are all factors. However, the one that strikes the greatest fear in us is cholesterol. If cholesterol were a Hollywood movie, it would be a blockbuster. The marketing success of health agencies in raising awareness of cholesterol has been enormous.

WHAT IS CHOLESTEROL?

Labeled as a "bad guy," cholesterol has been thought to play a limited role in the body. Contrary to popular belief, cholesterol has a number of essential functions in the body. In every cell of your body, cholesterol is a major part of the plasma membrane. The plasma membrane surrounds each cell and is involved in transporting nutrients, waste and messages between cells. Cholesterol controls the physical properties of the plasma membrane, which affects the function of membrane proteins such as receptors and transporters. Losing cholesterol in the membrane can cripple many functions of a cell.

Cholesterol has a second important role in the body. It is used to make bile acids which are required for fat digestion in the intestinal tract. The liver uses cholesterol to make bile acids. Cholesterol is also used to make steroid hormones such as estrogen, testosterone, corticosteroids and calciferols. As such, cholesterol is important to the everyday health and functioning of the sexual, mental, immune and skeletal systems in the body.

Eating a low-fat diet will not effectively lower your cholesterol levels. Your liver loves to make cholesterol, perhaps because it plays such a vital role in cell membranes. Thus, even if you do not eat cholesterol, you will have plenty in your body. Also, your body is very effective at absorbing fats. Your intestines are like a sponge for fats. The reason cholesterol levels can rise so easily in your body is that cholesterol is not used as an energy source and therefore does not get broken down as frequently as other fats you eat.

The liver is the major site of cholesterol biosynthesis. Once made, cholesterol is carried from the liver to all parts of the body. Cholesterol is carried around the body by lipoproteins such as high-density lipoprotein (HDL), low-density lipoprotein (LDL) and very low-density lipoprotein (VLDL).

Very low-density lipoprotein (VLDL) is the major lipoprotein made by the liver. VLDL transports cholesterol and triacylglycerol (another fat) from the liver to the other parts of the body. VLDL can change. If the lipids it is carrying are exchanged in a way that the density of the lipoprotein lowers, VLDL can become LDL. Low-density lipoprotein (LDL) has a high concentration of cholesterol. This is why LDL is commonly called "bad cholesterol."

High-density lipoproteins (HDL) are considered the "good choles-terol" as they collect cholesterol lying around in the arteries of your body and bring it back to the liver to be used in bile production. This is why HDL is commonly called the good cholesterol.

Why Is Cholesterol So Dangerous?

High levels of cholesterol in the blood are associated with an increased risk of developing atherosclerosis, a hardening of the blood vessels that can lead to a heart attack or stroke. In particular, a high level of LDL cholesterol is of concern. Atherosclerosis is the leading cause of death in Western countries; it is more common than all cancers and leukemia combined.

What Factors Increase Your Blood Cholesterol?

Diet, inactivity and genetic factors all contribute to high choles-terol. Consuming foods that are high in cholesterol and fat or eat-ing too many carbohydrates can increase the body's concentration of cholesterol. Sedentary lifestyles have also been associated with higher cholesterol levels. Cholesterol metabolism is controlled by your DNA. A defect in LDL receptors is known to increase blood cholesterol.

How Does Cholesterol Cause Disease?

It all has to do with the development of an atherosclerotic lesion. A lesion starts with a small tear on the membrane of a blood vessel. This allows plasma to leak into the muscle layers that lie beneath the surface of the blood vessel. The plasma contains cholesterol that triggers inflammation, which in turn causes damage to the tissue. A small, repairable tear in the blood vessel has now turned into a large sore (lesion).

Cholesterol also plays a role in the formation of clots at the site of the lesion. Clots are made by platlets, which are sticky. Cholesterol, cal-cium and other components of the blood stick to these platlet-covered lesions and can form a clot in the blood vessel. If the clot becomes large enough, it can restrict blood flow. This means not enough blood gets to the tissue downstream, and the tissue suffocates. If the blood vessel with the clot feeds the muscle of the heart, or is in the brain, the result is a heart attack or stroke respectively. But not every lesion will lead to an atherosclerotic plaque. Normally, the cells that line the blood vessles can prevent clotting.

Atherosclerosis

Blood flows through your arteries like water through a hose. Blood vessels (arteries) deliver oxygen and nutrients to organs, muscles and bones. When arteries become clogged with fatty deposits known as plaques, they lose their elasticity and become narrow. This blocks the passage of blood to the body parts that need it. This is known as atherosclerosis. The plaque is sticky and made of fatty substances such as cholesterol. The plaque can collect calcium and waste products. Atherosclerosis is a slow, progressive condition that begins in childhood and can occur anywhere in the body. It most commonly affects large- and medium-sized arteries. There are no symptoms for atherosclerosis and no direct treatment. Lifestyle changes are thought to be the best way to prevent fatty deposits in arteries.

How Can You Prevent or Limit the Development of Atherosclerosis?

By lowering cholesterol levels, you can slow the development of atherosclerotic plaques. One way cholesterol is removed from the blood stream is by cholesterol-requiring cells. Tissues that make steroid hormones commonly require cholesterol. These cells will remove low-density lipoprotein (LDL) from circulation through a process called *endocytosis*. Cholesterol carried by LDL can only be used by cells with a specific receptor—the LDL receptor. A genetic problem with this receptor is associated with high cholesterol levels and an increased risk of heart attack and stroke.

Another way cholesterol is removed from your blood is by the liver. Excess cholesterol can be transported back to the liver by high-density lipoprotein (HDL). A high level of HDL in the blood is associated with a decreased risk of cardiovascular disease. The liver can either recycle the cholesterol and make new lipoproteins or dispose of it in the bile. Certain foods are associated with an increase in HDL. Fish oil is one such food.

There are other ways to reduce cholesterol in the body, and current therapy usually involves multiple approaches. Here are some of the most commonly used therapies to reduce cholesterol levels in the body.

1. Limit dietary intake of cholesterol. Cholesterol does not occur in plants; therefore, your diet should consist mainly of fresh fruits and vegetables, nuts, grains, beans and seeds.
2. Increase good fat consumption. Polyunsaturated fatty acids found in plants and some animals, e.g., fish, support healthy inflammation in the body and may reduce inflammation associated with lesion development.
3. Increase fiber intake. This will help inhibit the uptake of cholesterol from the intestinal tract. About 95% of cholesterol in bile acids is re-absorbed in the intestinal tract and recycled.
4. Inhibit liver synthesis of cholesterol. This is how the pharmaceutical family of drugs called *statins* target high cholesterol levels. Red yeast rice is a natural product thought to offer cholesterol-lowering effects much like statins.
5. Limit the amount of cholesterol re-absorbed from the bile in the intestines. Probiotics can help produce enzymes that prevent this reabsorption of cholesterol.

THE PROBIOTIC CONNECTION

Elevated levels of cholesterol in the blood have been linked to an increased risk of heart disease. Results from early studies suggest that the consumption of yogurt, a natural source of probiotics, contributes to a reduced cholesterol level in the blood. A number of studies since have found that use of probiotics can reduce cholesterol levels by as much as 22% to 33%.

How do bacteria in the intestinal tract have anything to do with cholesterol? There are many ways in which probiotics affect cholesterol metabolism in the body. The exact means by which this occurs is not completely understood, but it is likely that probiotics lower cholesterol through a number of ways.

Probiotics may reduce cholesterol levels in the body by simply using or absorbing cholesterol. The bacteria cells themselves may use

Probiotics can reduce cholesterol levels by as much as 22% to 33%. some cholesterol in the intestines. However, it is a second mechanism that is more likely the cause of the decrease in cholesterol levels seen in populations that use probiotics regularly.

First, let's review the movement of cholesterol from the liver into the bile acids in the intestine and re-absorption by the body. The liver uses cholesterol to make bile acids (cholic and chenodeoxycholic acid), which are sent from the liver through the bile duct into the intestinal tract. A lot of the cholesterol in bile acids are re-absorbed by the body, and the rest are excreted in the feces (about 5%). If less cholesterol is re-absorbed from the intestines, then the liver needs to remove more cholesterol from the blood, which in turn causes a drop in cholesterol levels.

The ability of probiotics to lower cholesterol levels is due to their ability to produce bile salt hydrolase (BSH). Bile salt hydrolase is an enzyme that converts bile into deconjugated bile salts. Deconjugated bile salts cannot be reabsorbed by the body; thus, more bile acid is lost in the feces and less cholesterol is re-absorbed and sent to the liver. Since about 95% of bile salts are normally re-absorbed, this enzyme can have a great effect on cholesterol levels. The production of bile salt hydrolase by probiotics appears to lower cholesterol by reducing the amount of cholesterol absorbed in the gut and increasing the amount of cholesterol pulled from the blood by the liver to make bile.

In recent years, interest has increased in the use of probiotics to lower cholesterol levels. Researchers have screened more than 300 strains of bacteria for bile salt hydrolase activity. Bile salt hydrolase activity was found to be common in almost all Bifidobacterium and some Lactobacillus but not in *L. lactis* and *S. thermophilus*. Probiotics are a good addition to the diet of people with high cholesterol.

Some research papers suggest that probiotics lower cholesterol levels by inhibiting the ability of the liver to make cholesterol. Another paper suggested probiotics increase the ability of low-density lipoproteins (LDL) to hold cholesterol. It is not certain which way probiotics lower cholesterol.

There appears to be evidence that probiotics play a role in cholesterol management. Controlled clinical trials have found that probiotics reduced cholesterol in people with hyperlipidemia (high cholesterol). A crossover study of 29 healthy women, ages 19 to 56, found that the long-term daily consumption of 300 g of a plain or probiotic-containing yogurt increased high-density lipoprotein (HDL) cholesterol. The yogurt was enriched with *Lactobacillus acidophilus* and *Bidfidobacterium longum.*

A meta-analysis (a review of the existing studies to date) of six studies investigating a probiotic yogurt product containing *E. faecium* found that the yogurt caused a 4% decrease in total cholesterol and a 5% decrease in low-density lipoprotein (LDL) cholesterol. The connection between probiotics and cholesterol does not only appear to work theoretically but also appears to be supported by clinical research. Watch for more research in this area in the future.

Probiotics may help your heart by doing more than lowering cholesterol. A controlled, randomized, double-blind study involving 36 male smokers who consumed 50,000 CFUs of *L. plantarum* had a decrease in oxidative stress and inflammation. Thus, *L. plantarum* appears to effectively reduce some heart disease risk factors.

PROBIOTICS TO REDUCE BLOOD PRESSURE

About 50 to 60 million people in the United States are estimated to have hypertension (elevated blood pressure). This may seem like a big number until you realize that there is a 60% higher rate of hypertension in Europe than in the United States or Canada. Hypertension is a risk factor for heart disease. High blood pressure can cause strokes, heart attacks and heart and kidney failure. It is also related to dementia and sexual problems. Blood pressure is the force on the walls of the arteries as the blood circulates. When it is too high, as in hypertension, the arteries can become damaged and disease can develop.

Probiotics may help fight hypertension. Animal studies have found that Lactobacilli probiotics have a mild effect on blood pressure. This may have to do with the ability of probiotics to produce enzymes that break down proteins involved in blood pressure. There have only been a few studies looking at the effects of probiotics on hypertension, but the results suggest that probiotics may be able to lower systolic blood pressure by 10–20 mm Hg. The consumption of Lactobacilli, or products made from them, such as milk that is fermented by Lactobacilli, may reduce blood pressure in mildly hypertensive people.

Population (epidemiological) studies suggest that milk consumption or dairy proteins are related to a decreased risk of hypertension. Some intervention studies have shown milk products and dairy proteins have a blood pressure–lowering effect. Milk proteins are broken down by enzymes in your stomach and by enzymes produced by Lactobacilli. The broken-down milk proteins are called *milk peptides*. Several milk peptides have antihypertensive effects in animal and in clinical studies. It is thought that milk peptides inhibit an enzyme that causes blood pressure to rise, called *angiotensin-converting enzyme*. Milk peptides may also have other mechanisms to lower blood pressure such as binding minerals and preventing blood clotting. As probiotics are involved in the creation of milk peptides, having a healthy population of Lactobacilli in your body may help you keep your blood pressure low. Watch for future studies to test if probiotic supplementation can truly affect blood pressure.

The ways in which probiotics can improve your health have expanded beyond the intestinal tract. Although they seem promising, most of the benefits of probiotics outside of the intestinal tract are based on preliminary science. As for hypertension, the research is only laboratory based and has not been tested in humans.

SUMMARY

Hypercholesterolemia (elevated blood cholesterol levels) is considered a major risk factor for the development of coronary heart disease. Drugs used to treat this condition, e.g., statins or bile acid sequestrants are often expensive and can have unwanted side effects. Yogurt consumption has been found in studies to beneficially affect cholesterol levels. The probiotics in yogurt are thought to cause these cholesterol-lowering health benefits. Probiotic supplementation may play a role in reducing cholesterol according to preliminary research. Many probiotic species found in North American probiotic supplements and dairy products are known to have bile salt hydrolase, which is an enzyme thought to help lower cholesterol. The cholesterol-lowering effects of probiotics are not large, but are beneficial. The ability of probiotics to lower cholesterol is a benefit that can help us all. Probiotics may also play a role in reducing hypertension. More research is needed before probiotics can be used as an effective treatment for high blood pressure.

chapter
14

Probiotics and Cancer

A MICROSCOPIC VIEW OF THIS CHAPTER

- A healthy diet and your immune system prevent cancer.
- Probiotics eliminate substances known to cause cancer.
- Probiotics stop enzymes involved in the creation of cancer-causing chemicals.
- Prebiotics and probiotics have synergistic effects against colon cancer.
- Liver, bladder and lung cancer could be aided by probiotics.
- Radiation therapy side effects may be alleviated by probiotics.

■ ■ ■ ■ ■ ■ ■

Your body is made up of hundreds of different types of cells, all of which behave differently. A cell in the liver, although it contains the same genetic information as a brain cell, performs a completely separate role. Every cell has a map of instructions called DNA. Each cell is told when to reproduce, die and repair. When the instructions relating to cell multiplication and dying are wrong, the cell may start dividing uncontrollably and not die when it should. The problem then is every time the cell divides, these bad instructions are reproduced. The result is out-of-control multiplication. A lump or tumor develops as these cells grow faster than the healthy cells around them. As it continues to grow, the tumor builds its own blood vessels and becomes an uncontrolled entity in the body.

Why does cancer harm health and at times result in death? A tumor can grow to sizes that obstruct the ability of nearby organs to function. For example, a pancreatic tumor could grow to a size that reduces the ability of the bile duct to function. The result is improper digestion and poor liver function. Tumors can also produce hormones and enzymes that interfere with regular body metabolism.

The greatest problem with cancer is that since there are hundreds of different types of cells in the human body, there are hundreds of different types of cancers. The type of cell in which the cancer starts will generally determine the speed at which it grows and its resistance to treatment, although there are many variables involved. The location or type of cell where the cancer starts will give a cancer its name. For example, cancer developing from a skin cell is called *melanoma* and a cancer that starts in the lymph nodes is called *lymphoma*.

What Causes Cancer?

Carcinogens are chemicals that damage cells in a way that promotes unregulated growth and other cancer-like changes. The process of cancer development is called *carcinogenesis*. Cancer is a disease that develops over time and can be caused by any one of over a hundred causes. As such, it is almost impossible to determine the exact cause of cancer in a person. There are many factors that are thought to increase the likelihood of developing cancer. Here are some of them.

Tobacco Smoke

Cigarettes are arguably the most preventable cause of cancer. Cigarette smoking alone is directly responsible for approximately 30% of all cancer deaths annually in the United States. Why does cigarette smoke cause cancer? Tobacco smoke contains thousands of chemical agents, including over 60 substances that are known to cause cancer. Just to list a few, cigarettes include carbon monoxide, tar, arsenic and lead.

In 2006, researchers from the University of Florida discovered that cigarette smoke can turn normal breast cells cancerous by blocking their ability to repair themselves, eventually causing tumor development. In other words, the toxins in cigarette smoke prevent a damaged cell from making repairs to itself. This explains why smoking is associated with such a high risk of cancer. The risk of developing smoking-related cancers increases with total lifetime exposure to cigarette smoke. Also, **secondhand smoke** significantly increases the risk of lung cancer and heart disease in non-smokers.

Diet

Even a quick Internet search will indicate the strength of evidence suggesting that diet is related to cancer risk. As a sample of the evidence to date, eating soy, chicken, olive oil or using a low-calorie or Mediterranean diet are all associated with a lower risk of cancer. More than 30% of cancers are thought to be preventable with dietary means. A diet rich in a variety of colorful fruits and vegetables, whole grains and legumes is thought to offer the body many nutrients to help fight cancer development. What should you avoid? Alcohol, aspartame and barbecued meats are on the list of foods that may increase the risk of cancer. Want an easy rule of thumb? The more processed or artificial a food, the more likely it is to cause more harm than benefits.

Ultraviolet Light

The ability of the sun to damage your skin is well known. Sunshine is made up of ultraviolet light that can damage the DNA in skin cells. The sun's rays contain three types of ultraviolet light: UVA, UVB and UVC. UVA makes up most of the natural sunlight. UVB causes sunburns and is thought to be the main cause of skin cancer. UVC is mostly filtered out by the atmosphere of the earth and is of little concern to humans. Originally thought to be the main cause of skin cancer, UVB rays have been the focus of prevention efforts. However, new research points to UVA as a cancer-causing light as well.

The damage caused by ultraviolet light may happen years before a cancer develops. As such, avoiding too much sunlight is highly recommended. Who is most at risk? There are several factors that affect your risk from sun exposure, including how much time you spend outdoors, your natural skin color and use of sunbeds. Risk factors for skin cancer include:

- spending time outdoors
- using sunbeds
- having fair skin, hair or eyes.

As skin cancer develops slowly, you are more likely to develop it the older you become.

There are two main types of skin cancer: squamous cell cancer and basal cell cancer. Melanoma is the other form of skin cancer. Basal cell is the most common type of skin cancer; it tends to present as a bleeding or unhealing sore. It can look like psoriasis or eczema. Basal cell cancers are more likely in children with several episodes of sunburn in childhood as well as people with a history of periodical sunburns, e.g., holiday burns. Squamous cell cancer is slower growing than basal cell cancer but it is more likely to spread. This type of cancer is characterized by red, scaly skin that becomes an open sore. Squamous cell cancer is linked to an overall high level of sun exposure throughout life. As such, outdoor workers and those with epidodes of sunburn as children are at higher risk of this type of skin cancer. Melanoma is a malignant (spreading) tumor of the melanocytes which are found predominantly in skin.

Ionizing Radiation

Ionizing radiation is a known cause of cancer and other adverse effects. It is one of the most extensively studied human carcinogens and may account for about 3% of all cancers. How does it work? Ionizing radiation can remove electrons from molecules in your body, e.g., cell membranes, DNA, leaving them very unstable. The DNA in cells is particularly susceptible. Thus, ionizing radiation can change the molecular structure of a cell, which can lead to cancer development.

Where does ionizing radiation come from? There are some natural sources such as cosmic rays and radioactive substances in the earth's crust. This "background" radiation is a small amount. Medical X-rays used at the dentist to see teeth root health, X-rays used by physicians to investigate bone health and mammograms of the breast subject the body to radiation. Uranium miners and those living in areas close to nuclear weapons tests are exposed to higher levels of radiation. Ironically, some cancer treatments include radiation therapy to help kill cancer cells. Yet the radiation itself increases the risk of cancer.

Historically, radiation was used to monitor patients with tuberculosis. The high amount of radiation in the targeted area caused a drastic increase in breast cancer rates 10 years after this method of monitoring began. History has many examples of how radiation use is strongly linked to an increase in cancer rates. Atomic bomb survivors in Japan have increased rates of leukemia and cancers of the breast, thyroid, lung, stomach and other organs, illustrating another example of how radiation causes cancer.

In general, the breast, thyroid and bone marrow are most sensitive to the effects of ionizing radiation. Avoiding unnecessary medical X-rays is one of the best ways to reduce exposure to ionizing radiation. However, in many instances, the benefits of ionizing radiation as a tool for diagnosis of various diseases and as an effective way to treat some cancers outweigh the risks.

Alcohol

Alcohol itself is not a carcinogen. However, population studies show that there is a strong link between alcohol consumption and some forms of cancer. A strong association exists between alcohol use and cancers of the esophagus, pharynx and mouth. Alcohol may also be linked with liver, breast and colorectal cancers. Together, these cancers kill more than 125,000 people a year in the United States alone. This modifiable risk factor causes over 4,000 cases of cancer each year in Canada. Reducing alcohol intake could save thousands of lives. Current data suggests that nearly 50% of cancers of the mouth, pharynx and larynx are associated with heavy drinking. Although there is no evidence that alcohol itself is a carcinogen, alcohol may act as a co-carcinogen by enhancing the carcinogenic effects of other chemicals. For example, studies indicate that alcohol enhances tobacco's ability to stimulate tumor formation in rats. Heavy consumption of alcohol may increase the risk of cancer and is best avoided, as it has many negative effects on health.

Chemicals

There are many chemicals that have been developed since the beginning of the Industrial Revolution in the late 18th century. Each was created, as it offered a unique function superior to chemicals found in nature. Thought to be wonderful inventions, these chemicals were placed in everyday appliances, school buildings and foods. When they were found to be harmful to health, it was almost impossible to eliminate them from our environment. Despite the fact that the manufacturing of many of these chemicals has slowed or stopped, they are still present in our everyday environment, including schools, offices and public buildings. Here are some of the chemicals known today to be carcinogens:

- **Asbestos** is a crystal-like chemical that was developed to improve buildings. Today, asbestos is still found in the walls of many buildings. However, studies have shown an increased rate of lung cancer among workers exposed to asbestos. Those workers who smoke are at an even greater risk. When buying an older home, be sure to have a professional test it for asbestos.
- **Benzene** is present in crude oil and gasoline and is an important industrial chemical which is used in industry as a solvent or to make other chemicals and products such as dyes, detergents, nylon and plastics. It is found in everyday items including gasoline, paints and paint removers. Benzene is a clear, colorless and flammable liquid with a sweet odor. Research conducted since the 1980s by the National Cancer Institute has found that workers exposed to benzene, even at relatively low levels, have lower levels of white blood cells. Currently, the National Cancer Institute states that exposure to benzene may increase the risk of developing leukemia.
- **Laundry Detergent and other household cleaners** also contain chemicals that are suspected to be carcinogens. *Trisodium nitriotriacetate* (NTA) is found in many laundry soaps and is a suspected human carcinogen. Toilet bowl cleaners can contain *ethoxylated nonyl phenols,* which are suspected endocrine disrupters. *Silica*, which is present in abrasive powder cleaners, is a known carcinogen.
- **Phthalates** are widely used to make plastics and in personal care products. They are endocrine disrupting and medical literature suggests they may be linked to some reproductive defects in the male fetus. As many personal care products are targeted to teenage girls in puberty and women of childbearing years, phthalates are gaining

attention as a possible cancer-causing chemical that should
be avoided.
- **Pesticides** have been reviewed by European and North
American studies and are linked with an increased rate of
leukemia in children. *Atrazine*, a chemical found in household weed killers, is the most widely used herbicide in the
United States. It impacts reproduction in frogs. Atrazine is
banned in France, Germany, Sweden and Italy.

In a healthy body, antioxidants and a gamut of other defense systems prevent the number of carcinogens present in the body and work
to prevent and repair the damage they cause. However, when these
carcinogens are in the grass our children play in, in our homes and
in our rivers, it can be hard to win the battle against them.

WHAT PREVENTS CANCER?

Many food groups are well known for their ability to reduce cancer
risk: high intake of fruits, vegetables and flax seed (particularly the
lignan fraction) and consumption of cruciferous vegetables and garlic. As well, the consumption of antioxidants such as lycopene, selenium, folic acid, vitamin B-12 and D are well known to reduce the
risk of cancer.

Also, the microbes in your body and your immune system play
a role in preventing and stopping carcinogens from causing cancer
in your body. When we look at various populations, we see that the
consumption of probiotic-containing foods reduces the rate of cancer.
Animal studies have found that some probiotics can prevent or help
treat tumors. How do probiotics, the bacteria that live primarily in
the intestinal tract, play a role in cancer, a disease with a complicated
origin? And, how do probiotics help prevent disease in organs so far
away from where they live?

Knowledge to date in this area is preliminary. However, probiotics
appear to have three ways to fight cancer. First, certain strains of probiotics can eliminate substances that can be turned into carcinogens
and promote the development of cancer. Such a substance is called a
pro-carcinogen. An example of such a substance is nitrite. Nitrites are

unstable compounds or ions (e.g. NO^{-2}). Probiotics in the intestinal tract convert pro-carcinogens like nitrites into neutral compounds. *Lactobacillus acidophilus* is an example of a probiotic strain that can neutralize these problem substances in your body. Other species may also have this characteristic.

Second, probiotics can stop enzymes which help turn pro-carcinogens into carcinogens. Enzymes such as b-glucuronidase and nitro-reductase are capable of such action. These enzymes are secreted by bad bacteria, such as Clostridium and Bacteriodes, which are normally found in your gut. They particularly love to live in your lower intestine. With fewer enzymes to create cancer-causing chemicals, the body is less likely to develop cancer. *Lactobacillus acidophilus* is particularly effective at neutralizing harmful enzymes that promote cancer development. This may be the most important contribution of probiotics to cancer prevention.

The third way probiotics appear to have anti-cancer effects in the body is less direct. We already know there is a positive interaction between probiotics and our immune system. Probiotics support and stimulate the immune system in many positive ways. However, probiotics also help the immune system by lightening its load. Probiotics promote a healthy intestinal lining. This reduces the ability of bad microbes that we eat from entering into our bloodstream. With fewer bad microbes in your blood that your immune system has to trap

What Is Cancer?

Cancer is a disease in which a cell's controlling mechanisms are changed causing it to reproduce abnormally. A healthy cell has a built-in "programmed cell death," which will kill the cell when damage occurs. However, cancer cells turn off this cell-death signal. Cancer can develop in any one of the hundred different types of cells in the body. Cancers are named according to their location of development. For example, a cancer that develops in the colon is called colon cancer. If it moves to the liver, it is called colon cancer with liver metastases. Tumors can be either benign (non-cancerous) or malignant (cancerous). Benign tumor cells stay in one place in the body and are not usually life-threatening.

and eliminate, the less work it has to do. Your overworked immune system has less work to do thanks to probiotics. Thus, your immune system can focus on helping cells that are damaged and prevent these cells from becoming cancer. All in all, healthy colonies of probiotics in the intestinal tract can support the immune system, leaving it more energy and resources to focus on cancer prevention.

COLON CANCER

There is a wealth of indirect evidence supporting the ability of probiotics to prevent colon cancer in humans. Most of this evidence is based on laboratory studies and some on population research. Human studies will help confirm the ability of probiotics to prevent this terrible disease.

> **Epidemiological Study**
> Observing the trends in a population can also offer insight into the effects of a condition on health. These types of studies are called epidemiological studies.

When a population is studied, it is called an epidemiological observation. When scientists observed the frequency of colon cancer in the human population, they found that the consumption of fermented dairy products, mainly yogurt, may reduce the risk of colon cancer. This epidemiological observation suggests that there could be a link between consuming probiotics and a low risk of colon cancer.

The second most common cancer in both men and women in Canada is colorectal cancer.

The first time probiotics were thought to help prevent colon cancer was seen when different populations of people were compared and a difference in colon bacteria appeared to influence the risk of colon cancer. When Japanese-Hawaiians, North American Caucasians, native rural Japanese and rural native Africans patients who recently had a colon polyp removed were compared, the populations whose colons contained Lactobacillus species and *Eubacterium aerofaciens* had a lower risk of colon cancer. People whose colons contained bad microbes were found to have a higher risk of colon cancer. Thus it would appear that colons with lactic acid–producing bacteria (e.g.,

Lactobacillus species) have a lower risk of colon cancer. These good microbes must be causing positive health effects in the colon. Probiotics keep the colon healthy.

What influences the species in the colon microflora? A healthy colon contains a variety of probiotics, particularly Bifidobacterium. However, changes in intestinal microflora from eating a diet high in meat, high in fat and low in fiber; suffering from stress; or using antibiotics can result in increasing levels of bad microbes (e.g., Bacteriodes and Clostridium) and a decrease in the levels of Bifidobacterium.

Such a change to the microbes in your intestines results in an increase in enzymes that can turn pro-carcinogens into carcinogens, such as beta-glucuronidase, azoreductase, urease and nitroreductase. This creation of carcinogens increases the risk of colorectal cancer developing. Thus, theoretically by reducing the production of these enzymes by reducing the number of bad microbes in your colon, you can reduce the risk of cancer. In fact, animal studies have found that reducing the activity of these enzymes does reduce the incidence of tumors (cancer). Probiotics may be a way to reduce the presence and activity of these cancer-promoting enzymes in the colon.

Studies show that some probiotics can reduce bile salts, carcinogens and enzymes that convert pro-carcinogens into carcinogens.

Bifidobacteria probiotics may support colon health and prevent cancer development in another way. Bifidobacteria participate in the metabolism of various compounds including the omega-6 fatty acid, conjugated linoleic acid (CLA). CLA is thought to have anti-cancer effects. By helping the body work with CLA, probiotics can indirectly help reduce the risk of colorectal cancer.

Are there specific probiotic strains that are known to have anti-cancer effects in the colon? No, there are no known anti-cancer probiotic strains. However, specific probiotic strains have been identified in animal studies as having the ability to reduce the risk of developing colorectal cancer. *B. longum* and *B. breve* have been shown to prevent DNA damage by carcinogens. In addition, both *B. longum* and *B. animalis* can decrease the formation of lesions in the colon that commonly develop into cancer. *B. longum* may also have anti-tumor activity making it a great probiotic for defending against colorectal cancer. How exactly Bifidobacteria prevents colon (colorectal) cancer is not yet known. Long-term, extensive studies are required and eagerly anticipated.

Prebiotics may also help in the colon cancer battle. In the presence of the prebiotic inulin, *B. longum* appears to offer greater anti-cancer effects in the colon. Studies in rats have shown that when combined, *B. longum* and inulin reduced the formation of pre-cancerous lesions in the colon. In fact, the probiotic-prebiotic combination worked better than either one alone.

Perhaps the more prebiotics and probiotics the better? An animal study found that the probiotic-prebiotic combination of inulin, oligofructose, *Lactobacilli rhamnosus* and *Bifidobacterium lactis* (Bb12) resulted in a significantly lower number of colon tumors than in the animals not receiving the combination. It appears that a healthy population of colon microflora in the presence of prebiotics is a potentially effective way to prevent colon cancer. The symbiotic relationship between probiotics and prebiotics in the colon is well supported throughout research. Ensuring your diet offers your intestinal microflora sufficient prebiotics likely plays a very important role in human health.

Whether Lactobacillus species play a role in reducing the risk of colon cancer is not yet known. One lab study supplemented colon cancer–susceptible mice with *Lactobacillus salivarius* UCC118. The probiotic reduced the level of inflammation and the number of bad microbes (*Clostridium perfringens*). This does not mean that Lactobacilli can prevent colon cancer. More research is needed.

Can probiotics reduce cancer risk in humans? Experts are not certain. A prospective trial which is ongoing in Europe is called the European SYNCAN project. It is investigating the effect of *L. rhamnosus* GG and *B. lactis* Lb12 on colon cancer and may offer some new information as to how effective probiotics are against colon cancer. Evidence to date suggests that probiotics have protective properties against cancer. Studies have found that probiotics prevent DNA damage, which is an initiator of cancer. Some epidemiological studies suggest that consumption of fermented dairy products, which are good dietary sources of probiotics, might have protective effects against colon cancer. Thus, it is possible that using probiotics may be a natural way to decrease the risk of colon cancer.

LIVER CANCER

Liver cancer is the sixth most commonly diagnosed cancer in the world. Despite these figures, the cancer remains relatively rare, with 18,500 new cases in the United States every year, and about 3,000 in the United Kingdom. The highest incidences of liver cancer disease are found in East and Southeast Asia, particularly China.

Liver cancer is the third most common cause of death from cancer.

Hepatitis B Virus

Hepatitis B is a serious disease caused by a virus that attacks the liver. The virus, which is called hepatitis B virus, can cause lifelong infection, cirrhosis (scarring) of the liver, liver cancer, liver failure and death. About 3% to 6% of the world's population is currently infected with the virus and up to one-third have been exposed. Symptoms of the acute illness caused by the virus include liver inflammation, vomiting and jaundice. Vaccines currently exist for this disease. Hepatitis B virus is endemic in China and Asia.

Liver cancer can have many causes. The largest risk factor is thought to be chronic hepatitis B virus infection. Consumption of foods contaminated with aflatoxin, such as peanuts, are also established causes of liver cancer. As the liver is the site of detoxification, carcinogens are metabolized there, making it a likely place for cancer development. Of note, most peanuts produced today have low levels of this toxin and pose a low risk to your health.

To investigate whether probiotics may help prevent liver cancer, researchers from the University of Kuopio selected 90 male students from the Guangdong province in China where exposure to aflatoxin-contaminated food is common. The double-blind, placebo-controlled trial assigned either placebo or two probiotic capsules per day, each containing 50 billion colony-forming units of a mixture of *Lactobacillus rhamnosus* LC705 and *Propionibacterium freudenreichii* ssp. Shermanii. The administration of probiotics led to a statistically significant decrease in the level of carcinogens in the body. The reduction was 36% at week three and 55% at week five. When the probiotic supplementation stopped, the carcinogens reappeared. In other words, the probiotics lowered carcinogens in the body, which might protect against cancer development.

Additional studies are needed; however, it appears from this preliminary research that probiotics may reduce the level of liver carcinogens. Probiotics may be beneficial when unavoidable exposures to aflatoxin and other natural and environmental carcinogens occur.

BLADDER CANCER

Bacteria live on the skin, in the mouth and in the intestinal tract. However, probiotics can affect organs away from these common habitats. For example, probiotics have the ability to affect the bladder. In particular, probiotics appear to offer anti-cancer effects for the bladder. This is important, as bladder cancer is the ninth most common cancer in men and the fourth most common cancer in women.

Bladder cancer is the ninth most common cancer in the world and is characterized by a high recurrence rate. The bladder is a sterile environment and thus is not normally inhabited by microorganisms. How can probiotics help? Preliminary research in the ability of probiotics to reduce the risk of bladder cancer is one of the most fascinating areas of this field. More research is coming in this area. There are only limited results to date.

Researchers have found that probiotics likely offer a protective effect against superficial bladder cancer. One species in particular has been the focus of research in this area: *Lactobacillus casei* Shirota. This particular species was first investigated due to findings from an epidemiological study which found that individuals who consumed *L. casei* Shirota more than once a week had a lower rate of bladder cancer. The researchers found that the ratio for superficial bladder cancer was 0.46 in people who consumed *L. casei* Shirota once or twice-weekly and 0.61 for those who consumed it more than three times per week. In other words, those who consumed this probiotic more than three times a week had an even lower rate of bladder cancer. As such, *L. casei* Shirota became a probiotic of great interest in terms of bladder health.

Researchers took this population information into the lab. As a result of clinical research that found that the consumption of *L. casei*

> **What Is Superficial Bladder Cancer?**
> Superficial bladder cancer is a common term used to describe a tumor or mass of cells on the surface of the bladder. This type of cancer can be removed surgically with good success rates; however, it has a high recurrence rate.

Shirota significantly reduced the recurrence of cancer in the bladder. In a clinical trial, patients who had been treated for superficial bladder cancer were given *L. casei* Shirota with positive results. *L. casei* Shirota is not thought to inhabit the bladder as it is a sterile environment. Its positive effect on the bladder occurs in the intestinal tract. The hypothesis is that *L. casei* Shirota binds compounds in the intestine that can cause cancer, making them unavailable, thus they cannot be absorbed into the blood, filtered by the kidneys and sent to the bladder where they cause damage. Once absorbed these cancer-causing compounds cause damage to the bladder tissue.

Do probiotics have a long-term anti-cancer effect? A year after the completion of this study, patients were contacted and researchers found that those given *L. casei* Shirota had only a 57% recurrence of bladder cancer, while the placebo group experienced an 83% recurrence of the disease.

Whether other strains of Lactobacilli or other probiotic species offer beneficial effects on the bladder is not yet known. It is likely, though, that other species offer beneficial effects to the bladder. Future research is needed in this area to determine what mixture of species can offer the best anti-cancer effects. All in all, it appears that probiotics are not just beneficial to the digestive tract but offer healthy benefits to organs not in the immediate proximity of the locations that the probiotics inhabit.

LUNG CANCER

There is no research suggesting that probiotics can reduce the risk of lung cancer or aid in its treatment. However, some research shows a connection between probiotic health benefits and a reduction in lung cancer growth. In September 2003, the *International Journal of Oncology* reported that treating lung cancer patients with vitamin

K2 slowed the growth of cancer cells. Vitamin K2, or menaquinone, is found in egg yolk, butter and fermented soy foods, and despite its importance in, cancer fighting it only makes up about 10% of Western societies' consumption of vitamin K. The other form of vitamin K, vitamin K1, or phylloquinone, is found in any green vegetables such as lettuce, broccoli and spinach, and makes up about 90% of the vitamin K in a typical Western diet. Vitamin K2 is the form that offers you the greatest health benefits. Probiotics convert vitamin K1 in the intestines into the more biologically active form called vitamin K2. As such, if you have probiotics in your intestines which ensure that vitamin K1 is converted into vitamin K2, you may reduce your risk of developing lung cancer. More research is needed in this area, but this is another example of how probiotics are more than just a digestive aid. Probiotics can improve the health of the entire body.

STOMACH CANCER

The number of people with stomach cancer has decreased in recent decades in Western society, but it is still a problem around the globe. There are two factors that play a major role in the development of stomach cancer: diet and infection with *Helicobacter pylori* (*H. pylori*) bacteria. The risk of stomach cancer is higher in those who eat a diet that is high in salted, smoked and pickled foods, which is common in areas of the world that lack refrigeration as a means of preserving food. Another potential cause of stomach cancer is *H. pylori*. This nasty bacteria will be discussed in full detail in Chapter 15. It is not known how *H. pylori* causes stomach cancer. First, it is thought that *H. pylori* might enhance the production of free radicals (unstable molecules in your body that cause damage to cell DNA and can lead to cancer), increasing the number of stomach cells that have DNA damage. Second, this bacteria may change the structures of stomach cells, such as cell proteins. This may help cancer cells grow by giving them the structural changes they need to invade and thrive. Scientists are not sure that probiotics can prevent stomach cancer, but their ability to fight *H. pylori* may help. In Chapter 15, I will discuss more about the ability of probioitcs to fight *H. pylori*.

RADIATION THERAPY

Perhaps the most exciting way probiotics can help fight cancer is through its ability to promote health in people undergoing chemotherapy or radiation treatments. In 2006, Russian researchers reported the ability of a probiotic called *Acilact* to improve the health of mice when exposed to ionizing radiation and chemotherapy. The probiotics reduced the ability of bad microbes from invading the intestinal tract. The mice also had improvements in the health of their blood and bone marrow (blood cells are greatly affected by radiation).

Researchers then wanted to see if probiotics could reduce the risk of radiation-induced diarrhea. In 2007, Italian researchers reported that "lactic acid-producing bacteria are an easy, safe, and feasible approach to protect cancer patients against the risk of radiation-induced diarrhea." This conclusion came from a trial involving almost 500 cancer patients who were going through radiation therapy.

Radiation therapy targets cells that reproduce quickly. This includes skin, hair and the cells lining the intestinal tract among others. Radiation causes a very immediate effect on the sensitive cells that line the intestines. The result is an unhealthy intestinal lining. Using probiotic supplements to repopulate the intestines can improve the health of the intestinal lining and prevent bad microbes from growing and causing diarrhea.

The potential for probiotics to alleviate or prevent radiation therapy–associated diarrhea is great. Patients undergoing radiation therapy suffer from many side effects. Probiotics may reduce the likelihood of diarrhea and improve the health of the intestines. This means patients can absorb more nutrients and have less intestinal discomfort and disease.

SUMMARY

Cancer is the second leading cause of death in developed countries. Adopting healthier lifestyles such as avoiding tobacco use, increasing physical activity, achieving optimal weight, improving nutrition and avoiding sun exposure can significantly reduce a person's risk of cancer.

Over the past decade it has become clear that nutrition plays a major role in cancer. It has been estimated by the World Cancer Research Fund that 30% to 40% of all cancers can be prevented by diet, physical activity and proper body weight management. Nutrient-sparse foods such as refined flour and concentrated sugar products, low fiber intake, red meat consumption, and low omega-3 and omega-6 intake may all contribute to cancer risk.

Many nutrients and food groups are well known for their ability to reduce cancer risk: the consumption of fruits, vegetables and flax seed; cruciferous vegetables and garlic; and antioxidants such as lycopene, selenium, folic acid and vitamin B-12 and D. Probiotics, the beneficial bacteria commonly found in dairy products, are also supported as dietary elements to reduce cancer risk. Probiotics offer anti-cancer benefits including the ability to reduce pro-carcinogenic enzymes and produce short chain fatty acids which create a healthy colon pH which is associated with lower risks of cancer.

The human body was designed to be able to correct mistakes or damage in cells. Programmed cell death makes damaged cells die. Also the immune system plays a vital role in cancer prevention. A healthy immune system with sufficient resources should be able to keep the body healthy. Probiotics are well known for their ability to support the immune system and as such are likely to offer some support in the fight against cancer.

Preliminary research suggests that probiotics offer anti-cancer benefits to the human body. The risk of lung, colon, liver and bladder cancer may be reduced with the help of probiotics. Lactobacilli species have been shown in research to have anti-cancer effects on the body. Other probiotic species likely offer similar anti-cancer benefits to humans. Prebiotics may also help fight the development of cancer, particularly colon cancer. The most promising research is the ability of probiotics to improve the health of cancer patients undergoing radiation therapy. More research in the area of probiotics and cancer is needed as the use of probiotics to prevent and treat cancer holds great promise.

chapter
15

Gastric Reflux, Ulcers, Stomach Cancer and Probiotics

A MICROSCOPIC VIEW OF THIS CHAPTER

- Gastric reflux can be due to a variety of problems.
- A bacteria, *H. pylori*, is a major cause of gastric reflux.
- *H. pylori* can cause ulcers and stomach cancer.
- Probiotic species can help fight an *H. pylori* infection.
- Ulcers may heal faster in the presence of probiotics.

■ ■ ■ ■ ■ ■ ■

It burns. It hurts. Gastric reflux, more commonly known as heartburn, is an uncomfortable problem affecting many adults. Gastric reflux is a condition in which the liquid content of the stomach regurgitates (moves up toward the mouth) into the esophagus. The stomach's liquid contents can inflame and damage the lining of the esophagus. This is because the regurgitated liquid contains acid and pepsin. Pepsin is an enzyme that digests proteins in the stomach, and as such it can digest proteins in the esophagus. Acid is believed to be the most harmful component of the refluxed liquid, although damage to the esophagus from gastric reflux only occurs in a small number of people.

HOW DO YOU DEVELOP GASTRIC REFLUX?

Gastric reflux can be the result of a number of factors:

- Gallstones, which can prevent the flow of bile into the small intestine and in turn can affect your ability to neutralize gastric acid from the stomach.
- Not enough acid production in the stomach prevents the stomach from emptying and encourages stomach contents to move up into the esophagus.
- Hiatus hernia—a weakness in the diaphragm allows the stomach to move up toward the throat—which increases the chances of gastric reflux.
- Zollinger-Ellison syndrome, which increases gastrin production, causing the stomach's acidity to increase.
- Hypercalcemia, which can also increase gastrin production, leading to increased acidity.
- Scleroderma and systemic sclerosis, which can reduce the proper movement of the esophagus (throat).
- *Helicobacter pylori*, a bacteria, which is commonly found in people with gastric reflux.

Many of these factors cannot be easily fixed. Acid production in the stomach can be influenced by the types of foods you eat, how fast you eat and how much you eat. Probiotics can help fight one cause of heartburn—*H. pylori* infections.

HELICOBACTER PYLORI: THE GASTRIC REFLUX BACTERIA

The gastric bacterial pathogen, *Helicobacter pylori,* is the main cause of stomach ulcers and a major risk factor for stomach cancer. Gastric reflux patients are commonly screened for *H. pylori* infections as this bacteria is a common cause.

Helicobacter species are the only known microorganisms that can thrive in the highly acidic environment of the stomach. It has a helical shape, from which the genus name is derived. *Helicobacter pylori* has a unique shape that helps it penetrate the mucus layer of the stomach. The helical shape also gives it superior motility in the stomach. *Helicobacter pylori* will live in many areas of the stomach. Its presence can result in the formation of an ulcer. An ulcer is an open sore which is unable to heal due to ongoing infection or inflammation. Ulcers in the stomach can bleed and cause other complications. Ulcers can also be caused by the use of non-steroidal anti-inflammatory drugs such as ibuprofen.

Are All *H. pylori* Strains Bad?

There are many strains of *H. pylori*. Some appear to offer significant benefits to their human hosts, while others can cause negative effects in your stomach. Different *H. pylori* strains have been identified. Each *H. pylori* has a different negative effect on your health, and each can affect different parts of your intestines. For example, in Western countries, a person with one type of *H. pylori* (cag⁺, s1a vacA, iceA1 strain) is more likely to develop ulcers in his or her small intestine than a person harboring a different strain (cag⁻, s2 vacA, iceA2). In the future, more knowledge of *H. pylori* strains could help to identify people at risk of particular diseases.

H. PYLORI AND CANCER

An *H. pylori* infection can cause gastric reflux, ulcers and cancer. How is *H. pylori* associated with cancer? One of the known reasons for the association is the decreasing incidence of gastric cancer in North America. In fact, gastric cancer has decreased 80% from 1900 to 2000. The incidence of *H. pylori* infections in humans has also decreased in developing countries where sanitation and antibiotics are used effectively. This drastic decrease in gastric cancer rates where there has been a decline in *H. pylori* infections is consistent with epidemiological links between gastic cancer and this bacterium. Consequently, *H. pylori* has been categorized as a carcinogen by the International Agency for Research on Cancer.

Of patients who are not taking non-steroidal anti-inflammatory drugs, 95% of the cases of duodenal ulcer will be due to an H pylori infection.

How does *H. pylori* cause cancer? Despite the direct causal relationships noted, researchers are not yet sure how *H. pylori* causes gastric cancer. There are two theories currently under investigation. First, *H. pylori* might increase the production of free radicals, which can cause damage to the cells in the stomach. The damage can occur to cell DNA, which in turn can lead to cancer. Second, *H. pylori* may cause changes to stomach cells in a way that helps cancer grow. The bacteria might change a cell's phenotypes, such as cell proteins, giving a cancer cell the structure it needs to grow.

PROBIOTICS FOR *H. PYLORI*

As it is a bacteria, antibiotics are the most common treatment used in patients with an *H. pylori* infection. However, as we've seen, antibiotic use kills good bacteria in the body, reducing your immune health as well as your overall health. In addition, antibiotic resistance is a major problem. Antibiotic-resistant bacteria do not react to antibiotics. A growing number of antibiotic-resistant bacteria has increased the need for medical practioners to find alternative methods to get rid of an *H. pylori* infection in the intestinal tract. Probiotics may be an effective way to treat an *H. pylori* infection. Or perhaps probiotics are a good addition to antibiotic treatment. When probiotics are combined with antibiotics there is an increase in the cure rate of the infection. As well, there is a reduced rate of side effects from the antibiotics when probiotics are taken concurrently.

Can You Take Probiotics with Antibiotics?
Yes, the evidence supports the concurrent use of probiotics and antibiotics. Antibiotics are effective bacterial killers. As such, they can rid the body of invading pathogenic bacteria. Taking probiotics concurrently will ensure the natural microflora is maintained, which in turn ensures the health benefits elicited by probiotics are still occurring—in particular, probiotics' ability to boost immune health. However, probiotics and antibiotics should not be taken at the same time, as the antibiotic may destroy some of the ingested probiotics. Separating their administration by four hours is suggested.

Most of the clinical trials that have investigated the use of probiotics to fight Helicobacter infections have found that probiotics have a positive result. The use of many species of probiotics have been investigated in people infected with *H. pylori*. Both Lactobacilli and Bifidobacterium strains have been shown to be effective against this nasty bacteria. As with most illnesses, no one probiotic species appears to be superior to others at eradicating *H. pylori*. Let's look at the science.

In a randomized, placebo-controlled study, *Lactobacillus acidophilus* was given to volunteers with *H. pylori* infections in addition to their pharmaceutical medications. The study reported an 87% eradication of *H. pylori* with probiotic use versus 70% in the control group. *Lactobacillus brevis* CD2 also induced a reduction in *H. pylori* in a similar clinical study.

Other Lactobacilli species have been found in studies to eradicate *H. pylori* infections in the stomach. *Lactobacillus casei* Shirota reduced *H. pylori* in about 64% of the volunteers in a study, compared to only 33% of those not receiving the probiotic. *Lactobacillus gasseri* OLL2716 was effective in two research studies at reducing the number of *H. pylori* in the intestinal tract of adults, but not in children.

Lactobacillus johnsonii La1 has been investigated in three trials. This probiotic can increase mucus thickness and reduce inflammation in the intestinal tract, which are both great benefits to your stomach's health. However, *L. johnsonii* La1 did not decrease *H. pylori* in the stomach in these studies. Its other benefits to stomach health may make it a good probiotic to include in a multi-probiotic species supplement targeting stomach health.

The Lactobacilli species with the most promise to treat *H. pylori* infections is *Lactobacillus reuteri*. In a clinical trial, *Lactobacillus reuteri* ATCC 55730 (*L. reuteri*) was given to 30 adults suffering from heartburn due to an *H. pylori* infection. Twice daily for 30 days, the adults took their assigned treatment of either **omeprazole** (a pharmaceutical that reduces heartburn symptoms) and *L. reuteri* or omeprazole alone. *H. pylori* was eliminated in the adults taking the *L. reuteri*, but not in the group only taking the drug. *L. reuteri* supplementation also reduces side effects of drugs used to kill *H. pylori* in children. In a cross-over, randomized double-blind clinical trial performed in Japan, supplementation with *L. reuteri* reduced the level of *H. pylori* infection by 20% to 30%. Additional research from Italy found that *L. reuteri* improved symptoms of abdominal pain, reflux, indigestion, diarrhea and constipation in people suffering from *H. pylori* infections.

Why is *L. reuteri* so effective against *H. pylori*? *L. reuteri* is able to survive better in the stomach than most probiotic strains. *L. reuteri* colonizes the stomach and upper duodenum, all of which are sites of *H. pylori* infection. Also, *L. reuteri* produces a compound called *reuterin* (3-hydroxy propionaldehyde) that kills microbes (an antimicrobial). Reuterin may prevent *H. pylori* from living in your stomach. *L. reuteri* also has a protein on its surface that allows it to attach to the same places *H. pylori* likes to attach in the stomach. This means fewer places for *H. pylori* to attach and grow. This is called *competitive inhibition*. It means that the probiotic competes against the bad microbes for the same things (e.g., receptor sites, nutrients, space) making it hard for the bad microbe to live in you.

PROBIOTIC COMBOS FOR FIGHTING *H. PYLORI*

Is a combination of probiotics better at fighting *H. pylori* than a single probiotic? In a study, a combination of *L. rhamnosus* and *S. boulardii* was compared to a mixture of Lactobacillus and Bifidobacterium strains. Both probiotic mixtures were superior to the placebo (no probiotics) at making people feel better and reducing the amount of *H. pylori* in the stomach; however, neither eliminated the *H. pylori* infection.

A combination of Lactobacilli has similar results. When another study used *L. johnsonii* La1, *L. acidophilus* LB and *L. rhamnosus* GG in conjunction with drugs, they were effective at reducing *H. pylori* levels in the stomach.

A probiotic combination containing *L. acidophilus* La5 and *B. lactis* Bb12 was shown to significantly decrease the number of bacteria and the amount of acid in the stomach in people infected with *H. pylori*. Again, it did not eliminate the infection.

Of note, a combination of a Lactobacilli and yeast was found to be better at reducing *H. pylori* than the Lactobacilli–Bifidobacterium combination noted above.

It appears that many species of probiotics have beneficial effects to the stomach and reduce the amount of *H. pylori*. Even in the presence of drugs, probiotics help treat an *H. pylori* infection. Which combination is likely best? Each probiotic species offers a different set of health benefits. Many species help fight *H. pylori* infections. It is likely that a combination of multiple species and strains of probiotics will offer the best attack against *H. pylori* infections.

H. Pylori: A Silent Infection

Some people are infected with *H. pylori* and do not know it. They do not show any symptoms of disease. *Helicobacter pylori* infections affect about half of the world's population. They are particularly prevalent in Asia. Although it is a common infection, it is not a gentle one. Ulcers of the stomach and small intestine can develop over time if this bacteria is allowed to live in the stomach without inhibition by probiotics or other treatments. The most drastic consequences of an *H. pylori* infection is stomach cancer. Obviously, individuals who do not show any symptoms of the infection are most at risk. Since reducing the amount of *H. pylori* in the stomach may reduce the risk of stomach cancer, adding probiotics to everyone's daily diet might help reduce the risk of stomach disease in people with undetected *H. pylori* infections.

Probiotics for Ulcers

Once an *H. pylori* infection is treated, the stomach lining can be in bad shape. Sores on the intestinal lining, or ulcers, can persist. Do probiotics have any beneficial effects in treating ulcers? Animal research has found that *Lactobacillus rhamnosus* GG can help stomach ulcers to heal. A daily dosage of 10^8 CFU of *L. rhamnosus* GG for three days after an ulcer has formed can speed the rate at which the ulcer heals. *L. rhamnosus* GG is capable of living in the stomach, particularly in areas where ulcers occur. Research suggests that *L. rhamnosus* GG helps ulcers heal by beneficially encouraging damaged cells to die (**apoptosis**) and new cells to grow (cell proliferation), as well as by promoting the growth of new blood vessels (**angiogenesis**) to help the tissue heal. Other probiotic species may also offer some help in ulcer healing, but more research is needed. It is likely that these species will be of the Lactobacilli family as they naturally inhabit the stomach.

SUMMARY

Helicobacter pylori is a bacteria that likes to colonize in the mucus of the stomach. *H. pylori* is commonly found in humans and is strongly associated with heartburn (gastritis), ulcers (duodenal and gastric) and stomach cancer. Several probiotic strains, especially Lactobacilli, have been shown to inhibit *H. pylori* growth and infection in the stomach. Many species of Lactobacilli appear to cause beneficial effects in individuals infected by *H. pylori*. The most promising results come from *L. reuteri*, which was shown to completely eliminate the infection. A diversity of species and strains may be most effective in treating an *H. pylori* infection. *Lactobacillus rhamnosus* GG may help stomach ulcers to heal, but more research is needed in this area.

PART

Safety, Products and the Future of Probiotics

chapter
16

The Future of Probiotics: Superbugs, Asthma, Oral Health and More

A MICROSCOPIC VIEW OF THIS CHAPTER

- Superbugs are antibiotic-resistant microbes.
- Superbugs *C. difficile* and *Staphylococcus aureus* may be aided with probiotics.
- Asthma is immune-related, and thus may be prevented and supported by probiotics.
- Cavities and oral disease may be prevented with probiotics.
- You can fight the common cold with probiotics.
- Probiotics may positively affect mental health.
- Probiotics have detoxification benefits.
- Engineering may make probiotics into an HIV protection agent.
- Probiotics can be carriers of treatments.
- Some probiotics may help promote youthful skin.
- Kidney stones may be prevented with probiotics.
- Current research focuses on mechanisms of action.
- New probiotic species are likely to be discovered in the future.

■ ■ ■ ■ ■ ■ ■

In a world that can create an artificial heart and create machines with highly advanced brains, it is difficult to grasp the lack of understanding we have of the intestinal tract's environment. Probiotics and their relationship with the human body are complex and intriguing. There is much yet to learn in this area.

The future of probiotic research is promising and exciting. Probiotics are well known for their ability to boost immunity, prevent diarrhea and aid intestinal ailments. However, their ability to fight superbugs such as *Clostridium difficile (C. difficile)*, help with asthma and play a role in mood, detoxification and HIV treatment are areas of research to watch for in the future.

SUPERBUGS

Superbugs are not caped, crime-fighting bacteria found in comic books. They are antibiotic-resistant bacteria that are causing havoc in today's medical system. Why? Because antibiotics cannot kill these superbugs. Antibiotic-resistant infections kill as many as 8,000 patients each year in Canada and cost the health-care system at least $100 million annually. In the United States the figures are even higher at 99,000 deaths each year due to antibiotic-resistant infections.

A study by the Canadian Intensive Care Unit Surveillance found some startling results about the growing problem of superbugs in today's society:

- On average, 20%, and as many as 50% of *Staphylococcus aureus* (Staph A) infections in critically ill patients, are now resistant to commonly used antibiotics. Staph A can cause pneumonia and infections of the skin, blood, heart and bone.
- One in 20 *E. coli* infections in intensive care unit (ICU) patients is now virtually untreatable.
- About 7% of people ill with Enterococci infections have vancomicin-resistant Enterococci, which can cause urinary tract, wound and blood infections.
- Nearly 5% of *E. coli* infections are comprised of bacteria that are resistant to multiple drugs.

There are three superbugs causing problems in society that might be treatable with the help of probiotics:

- *Staphylococcus aureus*
- Vancomycin-resistant Enterococci
- *Clostridium difficile.*

Across North America and other parts of the world, these super-bugs are causing severe illness and in some cases death. Probiotics have antimicrobial activity, which means they can prevent the infection and growth of bad microbes, including superbugs, in the body. Some experts hypothesize that probiotic therapy can help in the prevention or treatment of superbug infections.

Staphylococcus aureus (Staph)

Decades ago, a strain of Staphylococci (Staph) emerged in hospitals, which was resistant to the broad-spectrum antibiotics commonly used to treat it. Called methicillin-resistant *Staphylococcus aureus* (MRSA), it was one of the first germs to outwit most drugs. This infection can be fatal.

About one-third of us have staph bacteria living on our skin or in our nose. People with Staph are called colonized, or not infected, as they have no illness from this bacteria. Healthy people can be colonized with MRSA and have no ill effects. The problem is that while they may not be ill, they can pass the germ to others who can become very ill with infection.

Staph bacteria are generally harmless unless they enter the body through a cut or other wound. In healthy people the result is minor, but in people who are elderly, ill or have weakened immunity, ordinary Staph infections can cause serious illness, including meningitis, endocarditis, toxic shock syndrome and septicemia.

In the 1990s, a type of MRSA appeared in the wider community. Today, that form of Staph, known as community-associated MRSA, or CA-MRSA, is responsible for many serious infections of the skin and other soft tissues and a serious form of pneumonia.

How does Staph become drug-resistant? There are two ways this an happen. First, a *Each year some 500,000 patients in American hospitals contract a Staph infection.* bacteria like Staph can mutate so it can evade an antibiotic. Staph bacteria can become resistant to penicillin, a common antibiotic, when it mutates to be able to produce an enzyme which destroys the penicillin. Secondly, it is possible for one bacteria to borrow the resistant gene (section of DNA) from another bacteria, thus allowing it to evade an antibiotic. This is how Staph can become resistant to the antibiotic methicillin and glycopeptides treatment.

When penicillin was first introduced in 1943, it was not known that *S. aureus* could be antibiotic resistant. By 1950, 40% of *S. aureus* found in hospitals were penicillin resistant, and by 1960, this had risen to 80%. Today, *S. aureus* has become resistant to many commonly used antibiotics. In the United Kingdom, only 2% of all *S. aureus* bacteria can be treated with penicillin. It is a similar picture in the rest of the world.

To date, there are very limited studies investigating whether probiotics may have a beneficial effect against Staph infections. A laboratory study has suggested that *L. reuteri* may be an effective agent to use against this superbug, but more research is needed. As probiotics help boost the immune system and some species have antibacterial activity, it is possible that probiotic use during a Staph infection may offer some health benefits.

Vancomycin-Resistant Enterococci

Vancomycin-resistant Enterococci (VRE) is a growing concern in today's medical system. The bacterial family of Enterococcus includes the species *E. faecium* and *E. faecalis*, which normally live in your gut. They usually do not cause illness in healthy people.

The first reports of VRE came in 1988. Today, VRE strains account for approximately 15% of Enterococcal strains commonly found; some institutions report an even higher prevalence. Infections from VRE are aggressive and have been associated with death rates approaching 60% to 70%. They are now the second leading cause of non-hospital infections in the United States, and the rate is increasing. Approximately 90% of VRE infections are caused by *E. faecium*.

What risk factors increase the likelihood of developing a VRE infection? Prior use of vancomycin, teicoplanin or other broad-spectrum antibiotics, undergoing invasive procedures, prolonged hospital stays, or being immunocompromised are factors that increase the risk of developing a VRE infection. The greatest risk is posed by exposure to VRE-contaminated objects or individuals, while you are experiencing any of the above circumstances.

Why are VRE strains so infectious? They have the ability to survive on dry surfaces for up to four months. VRE has been recovered from various hospital equipment (intravenous pumps, electrocardiogram monitors, bedside tables, blood pressure cuffs, rectal thermometers, stethoscopes and door knobs). This bacteria sticks around and it is a very dangerous bacteria. This superbug tends to receive less media attention than its counterparts—Staph and *C. difficile*. This may explain why research on ways to battle VRE infections, including the use of probiotics, is lacking. However, probiotics have some ability to stop the growth of bad microbes in the intestines, so there is a possibility that they may help fight this superbug. Keep your eyes open for more research in this area in the future.

Clostridium difficile

Of the three superbugs, only one has been treated in clinical trials with probiotics. *Clostridium difficile*, commonly called *C. difficile*, is a bacteria that causes diarrhea and other serious intestinal conditions. It is the most common cause of infectious diarrhea in hospitalized patients in the industrialized world. It was responsible for 108 deaths during a six-month period in the province of Quebec. While many of these patients were seniors and other factors contributed to their deaths, younger patients were also affected. Patients on antibiotics, with other illnesses and the elderly are the most commonly affected— healthy people are not usually vulnerable to *C. difficile* infections. According to the Center for Disease Control, 178,000 patients had *C. difficile* in 2003, which was double the number of patients with this infection in 1996.

An infection of *C. difficile* causes symptoms of watery diarrhea, fever, loss of appetite, nausea, and/or abdominal

Since 2003, C. difficile infections have killed more than 600 people in Quebec alone, most of them elderly or very sick patients.

pain. Diarrhea can lead to serious complications, including dehydration and colitis. It is considered rare but, as seen in Quebec, a *C. difficile* infection can be fatal. The standard drugs to treat *Clostridium difficile* are metronidazole and vancomycin. Although these drugs are successful in 80% of cases, about 20% of patients suffer from recurrence.

How do you develop a *C. difficile* infection? *C. difficile* bacteria are found in human feces. You can become infected by touching surfaces that are contaminated with fecal traces and then touching your mouth or nose. The use of antibiotics increases the chances of developing *C. difficile* diarrhea because antibiotics reduce the amount of probiotics in the intestines and colon which normally restrict the growth of bad bacteria. A decline in probiotics allows *C. difficile* to thrive and produce toxins that cause diarrhea. When you have the combination of a number of patients on antibiotics and the presence of *C. difficile* bacteria, such as in hospitals and long-term care centers, it can lead to frequent outbreaks of this superbug.

Probiotics and *C. difficile*

The ability of probiotics to help stop diarrhea caused by bad bacteria is well documented and discussed in Chapter 6. You will recall that when all of the double-blind, randomized, placebo-controlled trials were reviewed probiotics, given in combination with antibiotics, were found to be effective in treating bacteria-related diarrhea. In particular, the yeast, *Saccharomyces boulardii* and Lactobacilli species were found to be very effective. Of particular interest, was a study by McFarland and associates, which found that *S. boulardii* reduced diarrhea that was associated with antibiotic use. Plus, this probiotic prevented recurrent *C. difficile* infections, when given in combination with an antibiotic. Thus, probiotics, in combination with antibiotics, may offer some added benefit in preventing recurrent *C. difficile* infections.

Other types of studies, called observational studies, have also found that probiotics help fight *C. difficile*. There may be some benefit to *L. rhamnosus* GG, *L. plantarum* and *S. boulardii* supplementation during *C. difficile*-related infections. However, observational studies do not provide sufficiently strong evidence to recommend these probiotics as treatment options.

A laboratory study tried to identify which species of probiotics were most effective against *C. difficile*. It found that five probiotic species were effective against all forms of *C. difficile,* including *S. boulardii, Lactobacillus GG and L. reuteri.* These species may offer some help to patients suffering from an infection caused by *C. difficile.* Let's take a closer look at these species and the science supporting their use in *C. difficile* infections.

C. Difficile and the Elderly

C. difficile is a particular problem for the elderly. The elderly are at a greater risk of infection with *C. difficile* and as we age, our natural levels of Bifidobacteria decrease. Bifidobacteria are predominant among probiotics in the colon. Research suggests that an increase in bifidobacteria may interfere with the ability of *C. difficile* to cause illness. Bifidobacteria may inhibit the ability of *C. difficile* to attach to cells lining the colon. Studies on the effect of Bifidobacteria with Lactobacilli on *C. difficile* have shown positive results. More studies on the ability of Bifidobacteria against this superbug are needed before it can be recommended as a treatment.

Saccharomyces boulardii

This probiotic is a yeast that likes to live in your intestines. Two placebo-controlled, randomized control trials have shown *S. boulardii* is capable of reducing the recurrence of *C. difficile* infections. *S. boulardii* can make an enzyme that destroys the receptor site for toxins (toxin A and B) that is made by *C. difficile* and causes diarrhea. This may explain this probiotic's effectiveness against this superbug. In trials, subjects were also taking an antibiotic. Studies have shown *S. boulardii* supplementation to be safe when used by various age groups in multiple countries around the world. It appears that this species is both safe and effective against *C. difficile* infections.

Lactobacillus rhamnosus GG

This probiotic can help patients with recurrent diarrhea caused by *C. difficile*. *Lactobacillus rhamnosus* GG (sometimes referred to as *L. casei*) has some unique effects on the intestinal lining that helps the body fight against *C. difficile*. This probiotic helps stimulate the immune cells that lie below the intestinal lining. These immune cells destroy bad microbes on the lining of the intestines. *Lactobacillus* GG also helps the immune system by increasing the amount of immune chemicals, e.g., immunoglobulin G, interferon and other immunoglobulins being produced in the mucus layer of the intestines. This helps the intestines fight off infections. Perhaps the most exciting

ability of *Lactobacillus rhamnosus* GG is the production of a substance
that prevents the growth of *Escherichia coli,* Streptococci, *C. difficile,*
Bacteroides fragilis and Salmonella. *Lactobacillus rhamnosus* GG appears to have many ways to help the body fight off superbugs. Studies
suggest it is effective against *C. difficile* infection.

Lactobacillus reuteri

Lactobacillus reuteri is thought to be one of the best **antimicrobial**
probiotics to date because of its ability to produce reuterin. Reuterin
is an effective and aggressive antimicrobial. Reuterin prevents the
growth of many bad microbes in the body. Thus, *L. reuteri* is thought
to be a good candidate for superbug treatment. Laboratory studies
have found *L. reuteri* is effective at inhibiting the growth of *S. aureus*
but its ability against *C. difficile* is not yet known.

Prebiotics and C. Difficile

Prebiotics may also help with *C. difficile* infections. Prebiotics have
the ability to encourage growth of good bacteria in the intestinal
tract, which makes it hard for *C. difficile* to grow. Prebiotics encourage the health and colonization of probiotics in the intestinal tract.
About 10% of patients with *C. difficile*-associated diarrhea become
re-infected after treatment with antibiotics. Finding a method to stop
infections from coming back is very important. In 2005, British researchers found that supplementation with the prebiotic oligofructose
decreased the number of patients that became re-infected with *C. difficile*. Prebiotics may also offer some benefits to patients with superbug infections as they support the health and growth of the natural
microflora in the intestines.

Fighting Superbugs with Probiotics

What can we conclude about the use of probiotics in superbug infections? Preliminary research suggests that probiotics have the ability
to cause positive effects in the body, which can help those with superbugs to fight the infection. Whether probiotics can prevent or treat a
superbug infection is not yet known. Perhaps in the future, a specific
probiotic strain—a superprobiotic—will be found that can battle
these superbugs; however, to date, it appears that a diversity of species
offers the best benefits—no one species is a magic bullet.

Safety of Probiotics against Superbugs

There is some concern about the safety of probiotic use in superbug-infected patients. Studies have not reported any adverse events in patients with *C. difficile* infections who are taking probiotics. However, there is concern that treatment with probiotics may pose a risk of septicemia. Septicemia is a bacterial infection of the blood. When the intestinal lining is badly damaged and inflamed, as in some *C. difficile* infections, bacteria in the intestinal tract can travel across the lining and into the bloodstream. This is called **translocation**. Only one probiotic speices has been found to have the ability to translocate in research to date: *Lactobacillus* GG. Neonates may be more susceptible as one incidence of septecmia in neonates has been reported. The potential risk for this adverse reaction to occur is low; however, the possibility should be noted. More research in this area is needed before medical professionals will be able to effectively prescribe probiotics to fight superbugs.

ASTHMA

Asthma is one of the most common chronic diseases in childhood and one of the most common causes of school absenteeism. Asthma is inflammation of the bronchial tubes. It causes obstruction of the airway, chest tightness, coughing and wheezing.

If probiotics are primarily in the intestinal tract, how would probiotics aid the lungs and help to fight asthma? Remember that probiotics have a great influence on the immune system. Probiotics are likely to play a role in asthma prevention and treatment through their ability to moderate the immune response.

The "hygiene hypothesis," which was introduced in Chapter 9, explains the increase in allergic diseases over the past few decades. The hypothesis suggests that the increase in allergic diseases, particularly in developing countries, is due to a decrease in infections during childhood. Children are not getting exposed to microbes as much, and thus their immune systems are not maturing properly. The result is inappropriate immune reactions or allergic diseases. Clinical studies of children and animals show that being exposed to microbes in the intestinal tract helps to shape your immune function. In other words, an infant's microflora helps to mature his or her immune system and influences whether he or she will be tolerant or intolerant to allergens—the difference between being healthy or having allergies such as asthma.

The microbes found in healthy and allergic infants are different. Recent population (**epidemiological**) and laboratory studies have shown that a healthy microflora in infants helps them to develop tolerance to allergens. In other words, the immune system develops properly so it does not overreact—have an allergic reaction—to substances that we encounter everyday. Research shows that both asthma and eczema are linked to abnormal immune responses in newborns.

Can probiotics be helpful to children who are at risk of developing allergic diseases such as asthma? Finnish researchers have found that children who were exposed to probiotics around the time of birth were 40% less likely to develop atopic eczema than children in a placebo group; however, exposure to probiotics did not have any protective effect against asthma. *Lactobacillus casei* can reduce the rate of eczema in infants, but there has been no word yet on its ability to prevent asthma. *Lactobacillus rhamnosus* GG may exert beneficial effects on the development of allergic asthma according to preliminary research. The potential association between probiotics and allergic disease has prompted a wave of research in this area. Currently, there are a number of larger trials investigating the potential of probiotics to reduce the risk of asthma development in infants.

Trial of Infant Probiotic Supplementation to Prevent Asthma (TIPS)

TIPS is based on the *hygiene hypothesis*, which says that little or no exposure to bacteria and viruses during a critical period of infancy can lead to an imbalance in the immune system and result in diseases such as asthma, especially in high-risk groups, such as children whose parents have asthma. The study is investigating whether stimulating the immune system with *Lactobacillus rhamnosus* GG can prevent or delay the appearance of early signs of asthma. *Lactobacillus rhamnosus* GG is a common probiotic found in yogurt and many other foods. The three-year study will include about 280 healthy full-term babies whose mother or father has asthma.

An estimated four million children have an asthma attack each year and many others have "hidden" or undiagnosed asthma, according to the American Lung Association. The recent rapid rise in allergic diseases might be a result of improved hygiene and reduced family size. Recent epidemiological studies have yielded results both for and against such a hypothesis. The use of probiotics has a long tradition, and their safety is well documented. Prospective intervention studies in which the gut flora was modified from birth have yielded encouraging results. Probiotics may be a way to prevent allergies and asthma.

ORAL HEALTH

The balance between good and evil is as important in your mouth as it is in your intestines. A wide variety of microbes live in your mouth. Dentists are working hard to make sure we all understand that there is a connection between our oral health and our overall health. Probiotics play a similar role in the mouth as they do in the intestines. Below are some ways the probiotics are thought to promote health in your mouth. Probiotics:

- Play a role in protective biofilm formation on the teeth.
- Compete with bad bacteria in the mouth to prevent plaque formation.
- Use up nutrients in the mouth, reducing the amount available for bad microbes.
- Produce antimicrobials that prevent the growth and infection of bad microbes.
- Stimulate the immune system to work properly to attain and maintain health.
- Stimulate defense mechanisms in the mouth to prevent infection.

Probiotics inhibit bad microbes and promote healthy cells in your mouth. Since the health of your mouth plays a role in your overall health, then oral probiotics is an important topic in the future of this field.

A few studies have looked at probiotics in the mouth. In 2000, 130 volunteers in Thailand gave researchers a sample of the bacteria in their mouths. Over 3,000 microbes were found to live in healthy mouths. Five species were found to have the ability to fight bad microbes such as Candida. The effective probiotics included *L. paracasei* and *L. rhamnosus*. The study also found that the probiotics in the mouth were affected by pH, various enzymes and temperature.

Once probiotics were known to promote oral health, researchers wanted to know if supplementing with probiotics could improve the health of the mouth. In 2000, a group of almost 600 kindergarten children in Helsinki, Finland, were given milk that contained the probiotic *L. rhamnosus* GG for seven months. The children were between one and six years of age. The children in the probiotic group had fewer dental cavities than the control group. *L. rhamnosus* GG is known to live in the mouth for up to two weeks, which may contribute to its ability to improve oral health. In teenagers, a combination of *L. rhamnosus* GG and Bifidobacteria in a special cheese was able to reduce the amount of bad microbes in the mouth and support the use of probiotics for oral health.

The Elderly and Oral Health

The elderly may also get oral health benefits from probiotics. A probiotic cheese was given to 294 elderly people (70 to 100 years of age). They were randomly divided for this double-blind, placebo-controlled trial. The probiotics reduced the amount of Candida in the mouth and increased saliva production, which can be lacking in some elderly people. Cheese may be an ideal way to deliver probiotics to the mouth, as eating cheese prevents the enamel of the teeth from wearing (demineralizing).

The Best Probiotics for Oral Health

The selection of the best probiotic for oral health is an issue that calls for further study. Yogurt, milk and ice cream may also support dental health as they contain calcium and other teeth-healthy nutrients.

L. bulgaricus, S. thermophilus and *L. lactis* may also offer healthy benefits to the mouth. There is debate as to the benefits of lactic acid bacteria. They ferment sugars and lower the pH of the mouth, which are considered negative effects. However, they also have properties that improve the health of the mouth. Bifidobacterium species are also likely helpful in the mouth. Bifidobacterium species reduce gingival and peri-odontal inflammation according to early research. With more research it will be easier to promote oral health with the help of probiotics.

Prebiotics and Oral Health

Prebiotics may also offer benefits to the mouth; however, there are no studies on the effect of prebiotics on oral disease. There is every reason to believe that a prebiotic approach might also prove benefits to the mouth.

THE COMMON COLD

The common cold is the number one cause of absences from school and work. There are over 20 million lost school days every year in the United States from the common cold. The Rhinovirus causes the majority of cases of the common cold. Viruses cannot be treated with antibiotics, so the only way to fight a virus is with your immune system. Probiotics are known to improve the immune system in many ways. In 2005, researchers from Germany looked into the effect of probiotics on the common cold. They randomly divided a group of 479 healthy adults into two groups; one got a placebo and the other a probiotic combination of *Lactobacillus gasseri* PA 16/8, *Bifidobacterium longum* SP 07/3, *Bifidobacterium bifidum* MF 20/5 five times a day, at dosages of 10 million (10^7) CFUs for three months. When the researchers looked at the activity of these adult's immune cells, they found that those taking the probiotics increased the activity of their immune systems in a way that helped their bodies attack the virus infection. The researchers concluded that the probiotics significantly shortened common cold episodes by almost two days and reduced the severity of symptoms. Using probiotics for at least three months may help you fight off the worst of the common cold.

Probiotics seem to reduce the severity and duration of the common cold but not the number of episodes. In other words, probiotics can make the common cold less terrible, but it cannot prevent it. The use of both Lactobacilli and Bifidobacteria species is likely the best way to fight the common cold since having a diversity of probiotics offers your body a wide range of health benefits to help you fight this virus.

MENTAL HEALTH

They may not be the leading cause of death, but mental health problems are one of the greatest issues affecting the health of society. About 25% of Americans and Canadians will suffer from a mental health illness at some point during their life. There are many different mental illnesses, varying in their effects on disability, mental function and

Mental disorders are the leading cause of disability in North America.

age groups. This is a large and complicated health matter.

Probiotics and the B Vitamins

Probiotics do not reside in the brain and as such cannot offer any direct benefit to mental health. Nor is it likely that probiotics will be found to cure mental illnesses. However, some probiotic species are known to improve the levels of available B vitamins in the body. Probiotics can produce B vitamins, and these vitamins play a role in mental health. Ensuring your intestinal tract has a healthy flora of probiotics may reduce the risk of low levels of B vitamins in your body, thus promoting mental health.

The B vitamins are also involved in the metabolism of energy. B vitamins are required for the metabolism of carbohydrates, proteins and fats. In other words, you cannot make energy without B vitamins. Feeling energetic can improve your mood. B vitamins are a great way to boost your energy and feel great.

In addition, our mood is greatly affected by our intestinal well-being. When we overeat, we can feel uncomfortable. Consumption of contaminated food can make us feel ill and fatigued. Certain foods can make us feel bloated, unhappy and at times depressed. Ensuring your intestinal tract has a healthy flora of probiotics helps your intestines digest food, avoiding intestinal upset and keeping your mood positive.

DETOXIFICATION

Detoxification, or detox, essentially means eliminating toxins from your body. You can do this by having a healthy diet and lifestyle that helps support your body's natural elimination processes. Ideally, your detox diet and lifestyle minimize your exposure to toxins. It is kind of like stopping for a few days to do filing and tidy up your office so you can work in a clean, organized and more efficient space. Your body is the same. It is hard for your body to fight off disease when most of its energy is spent trying to handle a backlog of toxins from your food and environment. Detoxing gives your body a chance to clean out the build-up of toxins, giving you more energy to spend on more important processes in your body. Detoxing is especially helpful for people who are under a lot of stress, suffer from fatigue, or have a tendency for allergies, headaches or increased mucus production.

How Do Probiotics Help with Detoxification?

There are five major detoxifying organs in the body: kidney, liver, skin, colon and the lymph nodes. The main detoxification organ is the liver. The liver filters one-half gallon of blood per second. Responsible for filtering out all toxins from the blood, the liver plays a big role in your body's health. A lot of detox formulas will focus on the liver. Probiotics can help the liver too.

Research has found that probiotics can prevent liver and intestinal damage. When the intestinal tract is unhealthy, the intestinal barrier function can break down, allowing some bacteria from the intestines to enter the blood. The blood from the intestines goes straight to the liver to be filtered. Liver disease is thought to be affected by having to filter this type of bacteria-filled blood. Maintaining a healthy intestinal barrier is thus thought to reduce the risk of damage in the liver. Probiotics can help maintain a healthy intestinal barrier. More research is needed, yet it appears that probiotics may have a role in liver health.

Probiotics in the intestinal tract help to detoxify your body every day in two ways.

1. Probiotics are capable of inhibiting bad microbes in the intestines. These bad microbes produce toxins that can be absorbed by the body. Some probiotics can neutralize these toxins. This benefit can also be seen in the ability of probiotics to reduce the risk of colon cancer.
2. Probiotics can trap and neutralize other toxins, including heavy metals like mercury and cadmium. Exposure to heavy metals may have bad effects on human health, even

at low concentrations. Heavy metals can be found in our foods, drinking water and vaccines. Specific probiotics can bind toxins from food and water. Some species of probiotics can reduce organic mercury into its less toxic form. As well, some probiotics can trap organic mercury, holding it captive so it cannot cause you harm. By trapping, neutralizing and binding toxins in the intestines, probiotics reduce the ability of these toxins to be absorbed into the blood and cause disease.

Why Is Mercury a Concern?

Mercury harms the immune cells in the body and may play a role in autism. When mercury levels are too high, doctors will use chelating agents such as ethylenediaminetetra-acetic acid (EDTA) or dimercaptosuccinic acid (DMSA) to clear the mercury from the body. However, these agents are known toxins and can have side effects. Probiotics probably cannot treat high mercury levels in people but may be helpful in preventing the recycling of the mercury when the above therapies are being used.

Probiotics may play a helpful role in reducing the amount of toxins produced in the intestines by bad microbes and trap some toxins in the gut. All in all, probiotics likely reduce the amount of toxins in the blood and thus lessen the load on the liver. Probiotics may not be the most efficient way to detoxify the body, but they do offer some detox benefits.

HIV

According to estimates from the UNAIDS/WHO AIDS Epidemic Update, around 37.2 million adults and 2.3 million children were living with HIV at the end of 2006. HIV (human immunodeficiency virus) is the virus that causes the disease called AIDS (acquired immunodeficiency syndrome). The HIV virus may be passed from one person to another when infected blood, semen or vaginal secretions come in contact with an uninfected person's broken skin or mucous membranes. In addition, infected pregnant women can pass HIV to their baby. A person with an HIV infection can develop AIDS.

AIDS is a condition in which there is a weakening of the immune system. The effects are devastating, as the body cannot fight off common infections. Death due to infection is common.

Is there potential for probiotics to play a role in the prevention of HIV infection?

The number of people living with HIV rose from 8 million in 1990 to nearly 40 million in 2005.

Researchers are working with antibodies to HIV. Antibodies help alert the immune system of a foreign or unwanted intruder. If HIV antibodies are at locations where HIV contact can occur, infection could be prevented. Researchers have discovered that the antibody for HIV, a protein that binds HIV so it cannot infect cells, protects mice from being infected with HIV. In humans, HIV is most commonly transmitted during intercourse. Researchers at the National Institute of Health are working to combine HIV binding proteins to Lactobacilli. As Lactobacilli like to live in the mucus of the vagina, they are a perfect choice. Having HIV-antibody-carrying *lactobacilli* in the vagina may help prevent against this sexually transmitted disease. If these antibodies are present on the mucous layer, they could neutralize the HIV particles arriving in infected semen during sex. It has been suggested that if taken as suppositories or tablets, these bacteria could protect women during vaginal intercourse.

Despite the possibilities of this exciting new research, HIV infection is currently most devastating in developing countries where such engineered bacteria products would probably be unaffordable. An alternative strategy has been suggested: these probiotics carrying HIV antibodies could be grown in corn, thus creating "plantibodies." Corn would be a more cost-effective way to get these compounds into populations in developing countries that are at risk of getting HIV. Using probiotics as a vessel for antibodies is a fascinating new area of research and may offer a way to treat or prevent many diseases.

BACTERIAL FACE-LIFT

Very preliminary research suggests there could be a link between probiotics and the youthfulness of your skin. Bifidobacterial species may enhance the production of hylauronic acid in the skin. Hylauronic acid is involved in the elasticity of the skin. Two research studies have tested the ability of a bifidobacteria-fermented soy milk extract to stimulate hylauronic acid and improve properties of the skin. The results showed that there was an improvement in the appearance of the skin. Whether this is due to the probiotic or other nutrients is not fully known. Keep your eyes open for more research into the ability of probiotics to help you get a natural face-lift.

KIDNEY STONES

Kidney stones are one of the most painful of the problems you can have with your urogenital tract. Kidney stones have been a problem for humans for many years. Scientists have found evidence of kidney stones in a 7,000-year-old Egyptian mummy. Unfortunately, kidney stones are one of the most common disorders of the urinary tract. Kidney stones are caused by high levels of oxalate, a salt, in the urine. Probiotics break down oxalate that is in the intestinal tract. A healthy population of probiotics in the intestines can help reduce the amount of oxalate that reaches the kidneys. Certain species of probiotics are better oxalate users than others, according to laboratory studies. A half-dozen people were given a probiotic that successfully reduced the amount of oxalate in their urine, suggesting that probiotics can lower oxalate levels in the kidneys. Using probiotics to promote a healthy microflora in the intestines may help reduce the risk of developing kidney stones. The results of early research are promising, but it is too early to come to conclusions.

THE FUTURE IN PROBIOTICS

Researchers have gone back to the drawing board. We now know that probiotics are an important factor in human health. Having a better understanding of how they elicit these effects will help researchers better target certain conditions or diseases with specific probiotic strains. As such, researchers from around the globe are back in the laboratories trying to better identify the mechanisms by which probiotic strains affect the body.

Probiotics' effects are specific to their strain. In other words, the actions of one strain may not be the same as a similar yet different strain. For example, a mechanism preformed by *L. acidophilus*-122 cannot be extrapolated to the Lactobacillus species as a whole nor to all *L. acidophilus* strains. Each probiotic strain needs to be investigated as each may have its own health effects. Understanding these differences between strains could allow scientists to better target specific diseases.

There are more probiotic strains which have properties that enhance human health. Researchers are trying to learn more about these other strains. There are efforts to develop probiotic strains that have an anti-inflammatory effect, as well as strains with effects on oral health and allergy prevention. These new strains will be the basis of a new generation of probiotics with targeted effects on human health.

Probiotics are known to help fight diseases of the intestines that involve inflammation such as colitis and irritable bowel disease, but these diseases are difficult to treat by conventional methods. Physicians use pharmaceuticals to stop inflammation, but this is not very effective. Researchers are working on using probiotics as carriers of anti-inflammatory chemicals which could target the intestinal lining. This would mean a more targeted way to control the inflammation in these diseases and offers new hope to these patients.

The excitement surrounding probiotics is warranted. Like the discovery of a new ecosystem, the relationship between probiotics and human health is complicated—it's a whole new world to discover. Over the next decade, more research will open our eyes to the benefits of probiotics and the possibilities they hold. Your interest in this field is shared with millions around the world. Probiotics may soon prove to be the biggest health discovery of the twenty-first century.

SUMMARY

Probiotics have a bright future. There are so many things to still learn about probiotics. Research is looking at the ability of probiotics to fight superbugs, help prevent HIV, prevent and treat asthma, and improve oral health. These helpful microbes may also play a role in your mental health, detoxification of your body as well as help you fight kidney stones and the common cold, and improve and maintain youthful-looking skin. There is a great excitement among the scientific world about probiotics. Researchers are discovering new probiotic strains, more about what strains do and new ways to use probiotics to help human health. These microbes seem to offer many health benefits to humans. Perhaps probiotics can prevent and cure diseases that have troubled researchers for decades. Perhaps they will not. Only time will tell. In the meantime, the many known health benefits of probiotics make them a great addition to every person's diet.

chapter
17
The Safety of Probiotics

A MICROSCOPIC VIEW OF THIS CHAPTER

- Probiotics are safe for most people.
- Research studies have shown very few side effects or adverse reactions from probiotics.
- Many international research organizations work to improve probiotic research.
- Government food and supplement agencies ensure probiotic products are safe.
- Infants, healthy adults and the elderly have reported no adverse events from probiotics.
- Insufficient evidence is available to recommend probiotics to pregnant or lactating women.
- Probiotic use may pose some risk for immunocompromised individuals
- Prebiotics appear safe for all.

■ ■ ■ ■ ■ ■ ■

Probiotics are capable of enormous positive health effects on the human body. As researchers discover more ways in which probiotics can benefit health and they become used by a wider population of people, the safety of probiotics becomes of great importance. Labeled with the stigmatism of being dirty or bad, bacteria have an uphill battle ahead of them. Wish researchers luck in convincing the general public that eating bacteria is a good idea. Luckily, there is mounting research to support the effectiveness of good bacteria and other microbes in promoting human health.

There is extensive research available on the effects of probiotics in various human populations. This research allows us to come to a fairly confident conclusion regarding the safety of probiotics. Well over 500 studies have been conducted on probiotics and no safety concerns have been raised yet. Infants, teenagers, adults and the elderly have been included in these trials. Probiotics are safe for most people.

Probiotics are administered at what can be considered a very high dosage. The most well-known probiotics are of the genera Lactobacillus or Bifidobacterium, and most members of these genera are known to be safe, due to their long history of use and presence in the human intestinal tract. *L. acidophilus* and *L. casei* Shirota, which have been consumed for over 60 years are likely the species with the longest track record of safety. However, some probiotics do not have a long history of use. Probiotics used in most supplements and food products are species that have been shown in clinical trials to offer health benefits without safety concerns.

Based on current knowledge, it seems unlikely that Lactobacilli or Bifidobacterium pose any health risk to humans when consumed in appropriate dosages. On the other hand, some families of bacteria, such as Enterococcus, contain some species that are probiotics and others that cause disease (one is even a superbug). Thankfully, the species found in food products and supplements use researched species with well-documented safety records.

To achieve the same health benefits seen in trials you need to use the same strain and dosage.

If you are trying to target a particular illness with probiotics, be sure to use the same strain and dosages as used in the trials, as these are known to work. Scientific studies tell us that the specific strain, at a specific dosage, in a specific population of people works. Variance in any of these factors may produce different effects.

SIDE EFFECTS AND ADVERSE REACTIONS

Are there any side effects to taking probiotics? Orally, Lactobacillus species are well-tolerated by almost everyone. The most common side effect of Lactobacillus supplementation is flatulence, or gas. It is usually very mild and goes away after two to four days. Intravaginally, there are no reports of side effects with Lactobacilli probiotics. People who are immunocompromised should be careful with the use of probiotics as there have been reports of bacteria entering the bloodstream (sepsis) in these individuals.

Bifidobacteria supplementation is not associated with any side effects. In children, Bifidobacteria can occasionally cause mild diarrhea. There have been no reports of adverse effects from consuming Bifidobacteria in adults or the elderly.

Orally, *Saccharomyces boulardii* can cause flatulence. Rarely, oral use of *Saccharomyces boulardii* has been associated with fungemia (presence of yeast in the blood) in people who are immunocompromised.

Sepsis

Since probiotics are bacteria, they pose a small risk of causing sepsis. Infections associated with probiotic strains of Lactobacilli are extremely rare; however, translocation is possible. Translocation is the movement of a probiotic, which normally remains in the intestinal tract, into the bloodstream. It is possible for some species of Lactobacilli to access the bloodstream. In very rare cases this can result in sepsis.

Translocation of Lactobacillus
Scientists reported in 2005 that two patients who received a Lactobacilli supplement subsequently developed bacteremia and sepsis. Analysis showed that the Lactobacillus strain from blood samples was the same as the probiotic strain ingested by the patients. There are very few such reported cases.

A large study reviewed 89 cases of *Lactobacillus bacteremia* and found that immunosuppression, prior hospitalization, previous antibiotic treatment and surgery were common predisposing factors to *Lactobacillus bacteremia*.

The risks of probiotic use are considered minor. There are no reports of probiotics causing disease in people who are relatively healthy and have intact immune systems. Some immunocompromised people have taken probiotics without concerns. Adults infected with HIV were given 10 billion (10^{10}) CFUs of *Lactobacillus reuteri* orally daily for 21 days without safety or tolerance problems. Anyone who is immunocompromised should take probiotics with the care of a professional medical practioner.

DOSAGE

Clinical trials indicate that a minimum dosage of 100 million (10^8) CFU is required in most cases to see clinical effects. In other words, you need to consume at least this much to have a health effect. Some health conditions require slightly higher or lower amounts of probiotics to see benefits. Check the dosages used in trials if you are trying to target a particular disease with probiotics. Naturopathic doctors may be helpful in guiding you in the right direction. If visiting a naturopath or a medical doctor bring them your research as this will help them help you.

It is important to note that the body contains about 400 species of microbes and contains 10^{14} microorganisms. As such, there is no risk to your health in taking a highly concentrated probiotic. Available clinical data supports the lack of risk. Products are available with over 100 billion (10^{12}) CFUs per dosage. In Asia, probiotic products used regularly are of much higher potency than those commonly found on North American shelves and are used with no safety concerns. To date there are no reports of an upper limit on the dosage of probiotics.

INFANTS AND PREGNANT MOTHERS

Are probiotics safe for infants? Breast milk is a natural source of many probiotics and research suggests that the introduction of probiotics early in life is essential to the maturation of the immune system. Clinical studies have investigated the effects of probiotic supplementation in newborn infants (0-8 weeks of age). Both Bifidobacteria and Lactobacilli have been administered orally at daily doses of 9 billion (9×10^9) CFUs. Children (six to 60 months) have been given a mix of *B. infantis* and *L. acidophilus* at doses of 6 billion (6×10^9) CFUs per day. Both studies of oral probiotic therapy were effective in children suffering from diarrhea and no side effects were reported. There is insufficient evidence to conclude that all probiotics are safe for all infants. A review of the science to date and a discussion with a qualified health practioner is important when considering probiotics for young infants.

A handful of studies have looked at the effects of probiotics in pregnant and lactating women. These studies are discussed in Chapter 7. Probiotic species taken orally in a supplement or in foods can find their way into breast milk. There is insufficient evidence to recommend the use of probiotics in pregnant and lactating women; however, to date there are no known side effects or adverse reactions among infants or mothers.

THE ELDERLY

Many clinical trials have investigated the effect of probiotics in the elderly. This population is prone to intestinal problems and infections by bad microbes. Clinical trials to date have not reported any adverse reactions with probiotic use in the elderly.

PROBIOTICS FOR HEALTHY PEOPLE

Many probiotic strains have a positive effect on diseases, yet the current market for probiotic supplements and foods is not the ill, but the healthy. This is in part due to legislation in many countries that prohibits or limits the use of health claims on foods. This has restricted the ability of the general public to learn about the potential health benefits of probiotics and how they can be used to aid certain disease conditions. Probiotics are also heavily marketed to the healthy due to the strong evidence supporting the immune-boosting effects of probiotics.

Do Probiotics Enhance Health?

This is difficult to investigate because, clinically speaking, one is either healthy or diseased. There are no measurements for various levels of health. There are a few studies that support the theory of probiotics enhancing health in healthy people.

Children who were malnourished, but otherwise healthy, were given *L. acidophilus*. The childern showed increase weight gain and growth as well as a reduced incidence of diarrhea and fever. The researchers concluded that the probiotics appeared to have a health-promoting effect in these already healthy children. In another study, the effect of *L. rhamnosus* GG on children in daycare centers (one to six years of age) found the probiotic reduced absences due to illness, reduced the need to use antibiotics for respiratory infections and reduced the risk of dental caries (cavities). These healthy effects on healthy children were seen at relatively low dosages of 10 million (10^7) and 100 million (10^8) CFU.

Similar results have been seen with *L. reuteri* in both childcare centers and in shift-working adults. It would appear that probiotics may enhance health in the already healthy. Using supplements or choosing foods that contain probiotics may be a way to improve health, even if you are already healthy.

CONTROLLING SAFETY

The safety and purity of probiotics in foods and supplements is regulated in North America and so is not a cause for concern. As with all foods and supplements, there are government agencies that control the safety of these products. In the United States, the Food and Drug Administration is responsible for ensuring all probiotics in supplements and foods are safe. In New Zealand, supplements are guarded by the New Zealand Food Safety Authority. In Canada, it is the Canadian Food Inspection Agency and the Natural Health Products Directorate that ensures all probiotics on the shelf are safe. Other countries have similar regulations. Many countries, including Canada, require that all probiotic supplements are third-party tested to ensure they are pure, potent and of the highest quality. Foods are tested to ensure they meet label claims. These checks are helpful in ensuring probiotics are safe. In addition, the researchers involved in the production of probiotics for consumption strive to create the purest products. It is not in the interest of manufacturers to disregard the strict regulations that ensure probiotics are safe, as these products are sold on their health benefits— a bad batch would be a devastating blow to their sales.

There are a number of research groups around the world that are working to improve our knowledge of probiotics. The International Probiotic Association, the International Scientific Association for

Probiotics and Prebiotics, the European Probiotic Association and a non-profit group called the United States Probiotic Organization are just a few. These groups work with scientists, regulations officers and manufacturers to increase the knowledge of probiotics and improve manufacturing practices.

PREBIOTICS

Prebiotics are present in many foods we eat daily. Vegetables, fruits and nuts are all sources of these non-digestible fibers. As these fibers are found in our daily food, their safety is well supported. Prebiotics are safe. There are no reports of side effects or adverse reactions in people taking prebiotics.

SUMMARY

Probiotics have been consumed for years and use of probiotic supplements has generally been safe. Probiotic-rich foods have been on the market since before World War II without concern for health in the general public. Many research trials have found probiotics are effective and safe in a wide variety of disease conditions. In healthy infants and adults the risk is negligible. The only side effect of Lactobacilli and Bifidobacteria reported is flatulence (gas). Probiotics have been used in the elderly (up to 100 years of age) and in newborn infants without reports of adverse reactions. The use of probiotics in newborns should be done with supervison until more research can conclusively promote its use. Little research has been done on pregnant and lactating women, but of what has been reported there are no side effects known to date. There are some concerns of the possibility of sepsis in immunocompromised individuals and these people should use probiotics with medical supervision. Organizations around the world are working to improve the knowledge of probiotics so they can be used to effectively improve health. Government agencies around the globe ensure the safety of probiotic supplements and foods. Prebiotics are in our daily foods and are not considered to be a concern in any population group.

chapter
18

Finding Your Way through the Supermarket and Supplement Aisles

A MICROSCOPIC VIEW OF THIS CHAPTER

- Your health is most important. Probiotics promote health.
- Dairy foods, fermented foods and yogurt contain probiotics.
- New technology is putting probiotics in chocolate and cereal.
- There are five things to consider when choosing a supplement.
- Probiotic foods are more accepted than supplements and easy to use.
- Probiotic supplements are more potent, convenient and have better survivability.
- Getting multiple species of probiotics is best.
- Use the same strain and dosage as trials when targeting a specific illness.
- Regular use of probiotics is important.

■ ■ ■ ■ ■ ■ ■

There is potentially nothing more valuable in this world than your health. Take care of your health by offering your body the substance(s) it needs to function optimally. Vitamins and minerals are important for your health, and as we have learned, so are probiotics. Probiotics support your health in many ways: they boost the immune system, prevent infection from bad microbes and prevent and/or treat a whole array of diseases.

Do Healthy People Need Probiotics?

Probiotics may not be as essential to life as vitamins; however, there is mounting evidence that probiotics can help people stay healthy in many ways and may even elevate their level of health. Probiotics are also known to help decrease symptoms of illness and may treat or even prevent some diseases.

How Can You Consume Probiotics?

For as long as stories have been written about intestinal health, probiotics have been a part of everyday life. Caesar even mentions eating yogurt for his health. Fermented dairy products, such as yogurt, have been a staple in many cultures for generations. For centuries, many have believed that fermented milk products, such as yogurt, are beneficial to health. Elie Metchnikoff wrote the book *The Prolongation of Life: Optimistic Studies*, in which he noted yogurt as being beneficial for the intestinal tract and the promotion of longevity. Recent research has found that yogurt enhances our immunity to disease, may lower blood cholesterol levels, improve bone and oral health, treat immune-related diseases and have many other health benefits.

Today, probiotics found in products are typically, but not always, chosen because they normally inhabit the human intestinal tract and are known to be safe. Some probiotics offer you health benefits, but they do not colonize (live) in your intestinal tract. These probiotics are called transient but are still important to your health. Appendix 18-1 indicates the origins of some probiotic species. Species of human origin are thought to be more likely to live in your intestines; however, just because a probiotic was originally found in animal or breast milk does not mean that it cannot also be found living in the human intestines.

Probiotics are available in three different types of products:

1. As a culture concentrate added to a food (usually a dairy product)
2. Grown into a milk-based food and fermented food

3. Concentrated and dried as cells and packaged as dietary supplements such as powders, capsules or tablets.

Advances in technology are branching out from these traditional three forms of probiotics. Today, probiotics can be placed in a wide variety of food substances, opening the door to more ways for you to get probiotics into your diet. No matter what lifestyle, dietary restrictions or preferences you may have, there is sure to be an easy way to include probiotics in your daily life.

PROBIOTICS IN TRADITIONAL FOODS

Do you know which food(s) naturally include probiotics? Thanks to renewed interest in probiotics in the 20th century, more people know that dairy foods, such as yogurt, are natural food sources of probiotics. Lactic acid bacteria ferment milk to create yogurt. Many probiotics fall into the category of lactic acid bacteria. The acid produced by these bacteria curdles the milk and preserves it from putrefaction and spoilage. Probiotic species commonly found in yogurt include *Lactobacillus bulgaricus*, *Lactobacillus acidophilus* and *Streptococcus thermophilus*. Today, some yogurts also contain Bifidobacterium species. Yogurt can be a great source of probiotics.

Are probiotics naturally available in other foods? Some probiotic species are involved in the manufacturing of dairy foods such as cheese

---

How Much Bacteria Is There?

The amount of bacteria in a product is indicated by the number of colony-forming units, CFUs, on most packaging. Research supports that an adult supplement should contain 100 million (10^8) CFUs to ensure that sufficient amounts survive through the stomach and bile acids to colonize in the lower intestines. Supplements can vary in potency from 100 million to 100 billion CFUs of probiotics per serving. Dairy products such as yogurt with added probiotics usually contain about 200 to 300 million bacteria per cup. That's over 300 cups of yogurt to get the same number of probiotics in one high potency probiotic supplement. Supplements are the more potent source of probiotics.

and yogurt. Kefir is also a source of probiotics. Kefir is a fermented milk drink. It is prepared by combining cow, sheep or goat's milk with kefir grains. Kefir grains are a combination of protein, lipids, carbohydrates, bacteria and yeasts. The grains resemble cauliflower. Kefir, cheese and yogurt are all natural sources of probiotics.

NEW WAYS TO EAT PROBIOTICS—AND PREBIOTICS

Today, probiotics are available in all sorts of foods. The emergence of functional foods (foods with added nutrients that offer health benefits) into the marketplace has given rise to non-traditional probiotic food items. The easiest of food groups to add probiotics to is dairy products. It is not surprising that dairy products are the most popular food source of probiotics around the globe. Today, probiotic drinks are the fastest-growing food category according to AC Neilsen data from 2006. In fact, the North American probiotic market is projected to grow 37% between 2005 and 2010. Yogurts and dairy drinks with additional probiotic species have been well received by the public. Some probiotic drinks contain similar probiotic dosages to those seen in yogurt, while specialty products can contain up to 50 billion CFUs of probiotics per bottle. Depending on which country you live in, probiotic drinks will vary in potency, flavor and size. Yakult, Actimel and Muller are a few brands of probiotic drinks you can find in many countries around the world.

Probiotic-enhanced cheeses have also emerged in the North American market. Such products may seem novel to the North American consumer, but the concept of probiotic foods has existed for many years in Europe and Asia. A dairy-based probiotic drink, Yakult, has been on the Japanese market since the 1930s. China and Europe were first to introduce probiotic foods. Growing consumer interest in probiotic drinks has meant more probiotic products are emerging around the world. To learn more about the probiotic foods that are available, visit the United States Probiotics Organization. This not-for-profit organization publishes a useful website with up-to-date information on products available in North America. Appendix 18-2 illustrates some commercial food products available around the world and the probiotic strains that they have been fortified with.

Can probiotics be added to foods that are not natural sources of bacteria? If you don't like yogurt or have an intolerance or allergy to milk, then you'll be glad to know that many non-traditional food sources of probiotics are emerging on the market every day. This is a particularly active area. Advances in technology and manufacturing techniques have opened the door to a world of probiotic food possibilities. While yogurt and cheese have been traditionally used as delivery vehicles for both probiotics and prebiotics, other product areas such as ice cream, spreads and liquid milks are new vehicles for probiotics. Probiotics can be added to these foods by using modified species that are more resistant to environmental changes and the bacteria is put in a protective matrix to prevent heat and air from killing it.

Granola? Chocolate bars? Yes, companies have also launched both granola bars and chocolate bars that contain probiotics. In fact, Attune bars claim to contain 10 billion (10^{10}) CFUs of probiotics, consisting of the following species: *Lactobacillus acidophilus, Lactobacillus casei* and *Bifidobacterium lactis*. Why not skip the yogurt on your cereal as new cereals contain probiotics? *Kashi* has a cereal that claims to contain one billion (10^9) CFUs per serving of *L. acidophilus*. Meat products, teas, fruit juices and waters are examples of food products with probiotics available around the world. With the growing knowledge of the health benefits of probiotics, expect to see probiotics added to an even wider diversity of food types.

Prebiotics are also gaining presence on the supermarket shelf. Prebiotics can be found in breads, cereals and many other grain-based products. You can also find prebiotics in fruit bars, sweeteners and many other foods. Savvy manufacturers are adding prebiotics into their probiotic products to offer an all-in-one product.

What's next? Advances in technology and growing consumer acceptance of probiotics means anything is a possibility. The importance of having probiotics in your daily diet cannot be underestimated. Luckily consumer demand and innovations in manufacturing are creating easy ways for you to get them. What other probiotic products might be next to hit your local supermarket shelves? Only time will tell. As the supermarket shelves dawn new probiotic-containing products in the future, remember that sugar-laden products are still unhealthy for you. A chocolate bar fortified with probiotics is still a chocolate bar—a sugar-filled, fatty food choice with little nutritional value. Choose your probiotic product wisely and you'll enjoy healthy living.

PROBIOTICS IN SUPPLEMENTS

Walking down the supplement aisle used to frighten me. There were so many choices, species, potencies and marketing messages on the probiotics. However, the information provided in this book has made you an expert. You will surely find the supplement aisle a more pleasant experience now. There are so many different brands, products and species available in supplement products around the world. Remember that all in all, any probiotic supplementation is good. Manufacturers today use advanced techniques to cultivate and stabilize probiotics for safe and effective delivery in supplements. Nonetheless, there are certain factors you should consider when choosing a probiotic supplement. Considering these factors will help you find the perfect probiotic for you.

Potency

Clinical trials have shown that supplementation with probiotics is most effective when there is a sufficient number of living organisms ingested. The potency of a probiotic supplement is measured in colony-forming units (CFUs) of living organisms. For best results, a probiotic supplement should have a minimum potency of 100 million (10^8) CFUs or greater. Products can contain over 100 billion (10^{11}) CFUs. These higher dosages are good for re-population of an intestinal tract that has been severe changes in the microflora due to antibiotic use or diarrhea, for example.

As probiotics are living organisms they can die. Some experts suggest that probiotics have a short life cycle in your body of less than a week. As such, continual supplementation is required. Also, as probiotics can die, it is important to know if the manufacturer of the supplement ensures the bacteria remain alive. Ensuring your probiotic supplement is refrigerated, if required, will reduce any loss of potency. One manufacturer reported that its tests indicate that there is minimal die-off (only 7%) of the bacteria in a capsule after one week of storage at room temperature. Thus, if you leave them out or want to travel with your probiotic supplements, do not worry, as the die-off is minimal over the short term. New technology has created a shelf-stable capsule called a "pearl" which allows a probiotic supplement to remain out of the refrigerator for the duration of the product's shelf-life. These can be very useful for those away from home for longer durations.

It is also important to know whether the potency listed on the packaging of a supplement is the amount in the capsule/tablet on the date of manufacturing or on the date of expiry. Good probiotic manufacturers will guarantee the probiotic potency until the date of expiry. This means there are more probiotics in the supplement, ensuring you get lots of live probiotics to help you be healthy.

Age or Condition-Specific Formulas

Age or condition-specific formulas can help indicate if the species in the supplement is beneficial to your needs. Most probiotic supplements are made with strains that are commonly found in the microflora of the general adult population. Other supplements are formulated to help balance the microflora of a specific age group. The targeted age group is usually indicated on packaging.

Why would there be a need for different probiotic species at different ages? The composition of intestinal flora varies with age. From birth to old age, the species and concentrations of probiotics found in your intestinal tract will change. Let's use Bifidobacteria as an example. In infants, the Bifidobacteria (*B. infantis* and *B. breve*) are the dominant probiotics. These are found less frequently in adults. Instead, an adult's intestinal tract tends to contain *B. bifidum* and *B. longum*. As we continue to age, more changes occur. After the age of 50, the concentration of Bifidobacteria starts to decline steadily. Meanwhile bad microbes, such as coliforms and Welch's bacilli, increase. We start to experience immune system deficiencies and an increased incidence of cancer at the same time that our Bifidobacteria levels decline. The elderly also tend to suffer from constipation due to a lack of Bifidobacteria. Some probiotic supplements are formulated for particular age groups to meet these varying needs throughout life. For example, a formula for the elderly will focus on Bifidobacteria species, as this population is commonly deficient. Some formulas are targeted for children and as such will contain species commonly found in healthy infants including *L. rhamnosus, L. acidophilus* and *B. longum.*

Condition-specific formulations are less common with the state of current research; however, a few are available. *L. reuteri* is known to be effective against diarrhea and as an immune booster. Bifidobacteria are known to help with constipation and products with lots of Bifidobacteria may be marketed for colon health. Some products target individuals who have experienced digestive distress from using antibiotics, cleansing (e.g., detoxing) or traveling. Such formulas contain high potencies of multiple Lactobacilli and Bifidobacterium strains. Around the world, you can find examples of products that are designed for a particular health concern, but these are not very common.

Production Techniques

There are two main ways of making probiotics. In a sterile laboratory environment, probiotics are cultured under strict controls to ensure that purity and potency are attained. Bacteria can mutate and contaminants can enter cultures; thus strict quality controls are required. Advances in technology allow today's probiotic supplements to be guaranteed to contain only the probiotics listed on the label and no other bacteria or contaminants. Good manufacturers will note this on their label or in their marketing information.

More recently, another form of probiotic manufacturing has gained popularity. Soil-based organisms are thought to be a more natural way to consume probiotics. Some manufacturers are producing probiotics that are grown on soil and thus are marketing them as soil-based organisms. Historically, more bacteria from soil found its way into our digestive systems. This is one of the bases for the theory of why to use this type of supplement. It is important to note that culturing probiotics

---

Are Probiotics in Supplements Alive?
Inside those capsules are dried bacteria that despite most people's belief are alive! The microbes are simply dormant and stable. Refrigeration increases the stability of probiotics, particularly in dairy products. Follow the manufacturer's recommendation on how to store the product to ensure maximum survivability.

in soil limits some of the quality controls that can be implemented in sterile glass vials used to make probiotics in laboratories.

Survivability

Survivability of a probiotic may be the most important thing to consider. As most probiotic supplements are ingested, they need to be able to survive the acidic environment of the stomach and the basic (alkaline) environment of the small intestine. Certain strains such as *L. reuteri* are naturally able to survive the acidic environment of the stomach. However, the majority of probiotics do not have a high survival rate in an acidic environment. Thus, enteric-coating probiotic capsules can be important. Enteric-coating ensures that the microorganisms within the capsule will not be released until they have reached an alkaline environment such as that found in the small intestine. This is a great way to ensure probiotics are still alive by the time they reach your intestines.

Probiotic powders and chewable products cannot be enteric-coated. These products are best consumed one hour after a meal when stomach acid levels are at their lowest, or during a meal. Some probiotic powders and chewables use probiotics strains that are resistant to acidic and basic environments. Using these supplements can ensure enough probiotics will make it to your intestines alive.

Reliability

Is the manufacturer reputable? Reliability is also a factor to consider when choosing a probiotic supplement. If after looking into the potency, formula and survivability of a probiotic supplement you are still unsure, you can ask your health food retailer about the manufacturer's track record and commitment to quality. Websites are also a great resource for additional information. All manufacturers in Canada, the United States and many other countries must list a contact telephone number. Feel free to contact a manufacturer and ask them about these five factors to help you choose the probiotic supplement that is best for you.

TO EAT OR SWALLOW?

Historically, probiotics have only been available in foods, particularly in dairy products. However, with new technology, we are now able to identify a beneficial strain, cultivate it and get it into your intestines in large quantities. Research has used both supplements and dairy-based products in their investigations of the health benefits of probiotics. At this time, there is no true winner between food and supplement forms of probiotics. Supplements offer three unique advantages: they are more potent, portable (newer technologies allow for shelf-stable probiotics) and contain more varieties of probiotics which offer more health benefits. Meanwhile, probiotic foods are very convenient and can easily be substituted for other foods in your daily regime.

Both foods and supplements are good sources of probiotics. Each varies in its potency and survivability. A good supplement will contain 100 million (10^8) CFUs, which is the equivalent of about 300 cups of milk. Yogurt has more probiotics than milk and some specialized probiotic yogurts offer even higher potencies. Yogurts containing additional probiotics offer more types of species and higher potencies, which are both great assets; however, keep in mind that many mainstream probiotic yogurts also contain a lot of simple sugar which feeds bad microbes including Candida. In terms of potency, supplements may have the advantage over foods.

The guarantee that the probiotics are alive at the time of consumption is very important as we saw above. Refrigerated products are kept cool to reduce the chances of microbe death from heat. Check the date of manufacturing or best before date on probiotic foods. A yogurt close to expiry will contain fewer probiotics than one that was just made. The closer to the date of expiry, the lower the number of live probiotics will be in the food. Putting probiotics into capsules protects the probiotics from moisture and air when on the shelf. This means fewer probiotics die over the supplements' shelf life. Enteric coating helps probiotics survive stomach acid. Some new capsules even allow for supplements to be shelf-stable (called pearls in North America), meaning the probiotics are not vulnerable to moisture, air or heat.

Probiotic supplements are potent, safe and an effective way to introduce or re-introduce beneficial microbes into your body. Probiotic foods have a long history of association with health and they are gaining in popularity. Dairy products are already associated in the public's mind with health benefits to the body. Also, consuming bacteria in a capsule can be a tough thing for some people to accept. Yet, eating bacteria in dairy products is something we have done for decades and thus probiotic dairy foods are well accepted by most people. Marketers of new probiotic foods will have to convince people that eating bacteria is a good thing; they'll have to change the mentality that all bacteria are bad.

As you can see, there are benefits to both food and supplement forms of probiotics. But what about convenience? Capsules are easy to take, but they're also easy to forget. Probiotic foods can be exchanged for regular foods in the diet but can be hard to consume in sufficient quantity and frequency. Trying to decide which way you are going to take your probiotics may be tough; both have many benefits. The decision is yours. Regardless of which way you get your probiotics (food, supplement or both), know that they offer you many healthy benefits.

WHICH PROBIOTIC IS BEST?

This is probably the most difficult question to answer. It is possible that there is no correct answer. It is my guess that there is no perfect probiotic but that for health we need a variety of probiotic species.

Like fingerprints, each human's intestinal microflora has a unique makeup. A probiotic containing many types of probiotics will more closely resemble your normal microflora. This is likely the best way to take a probiotic. For optimal health you need both families (Lactobacilli and Bifidobacteria) of probiotics in your diet. Both have health effects for your entire body.

Do you need a simple guideline to help you decide which probiotic supplement is best for you? Simply remember where species like to live. Lactobacilli are predominantly found in the small intestine. Bifidobacteria are predominantly found in the large intestine (colon). For example, problems with the colon may be best aided with Bifidobacteria that like to live there. Yeast infections are best treated with Lactobacilli as these species are the dominant probiotics in the vagina. This is an over-simplification, but it can be helpful.

When considering which probiotic species is best for you, do your homework and find out what scientists know to date about your health condition of interest. In most cases, no one probiotic species is known to be the most effective for any one health condition. We do know that Lactobacteria all appear to promote a positive effect on the immune system and support digestion. We also know that Bifidobacteria support colon health and can help maintain regularity. As such, we can use these general points of knowledge to guide us toward groups of probiotics likely to aid our condition.

Once you've chosen a species, which strain is best? Each probiotic strain works in a slightly different way. For example, there are many different strains of *L. rhamnosus*, each of which in research appears to be similar, yet unique, in its behaviour. Luckily, species tend to have some similarities. Consequently, do not worry about what different strains do; that is too complicated. Only worry about strains if you are trying to target a particular disease for which clinical trials have shown a particular strain to work.

The majority of the research to date suggests that a multi-species approach is best. Taking a probiotic food or supplement that has a wide variety of species will better mimic your natural intestinal environment. We each might respond differently to different formulations. If you

Regular probiotic intake is important, as probiotics may stay in your intestinal tract for as little as one week.

Probiotic Origins

A probiotic's origin is the location from which it was originally isolated. For example, *L. reuteri* was originally isolated (removed) from breast milk; *B. lactis* from fermented milk and *B. animalis* from animal feces. This does not mean that these species have any characteristics of these locations. Bacteria and yeast strains found in humans are capable of colonizing in humans. However, animal-isolated probiotics have been found in studies to colonize effectively in humans as well. As such, when purchasing a probiotic, the origins need not be a major priority. Appendix 18-1 lists the origins of some species of probiotics. Various strains of a species may come from different origins.

find one that works for you, stick with it. If one does not work for you, try another.

One a Day to Keep the Doctor Away

How often should you take a probiotic for best effects? Based on clinical research, you will get the most health benefits with dosages of at least 100 million (10^8) CFUs per day. The higher the potency, the more likely the probiotics are going to arrive in their desired location in large enough amounts to grow and colonize. Whether a probiotic is likely to live in the intestines for a long period of time is uncertain. Many studies suggest that regardless of the probiotics species' origins, it may only stay in the intestinal tract for a week to 10 days. To receive the best health effects, it's important to consume probiotics on a regular basis. You'll recall that poor dietary habits, over-consumption of foods, stress, illness and antibiotic use can alter the probiotic balance in your body. Therefore, it's a good idea to use probiotics daily for optimal health.

Summary

Probiotics offer the human body a variety of health benefits. Your health is the most important thing in your life. Probiotics promote health. You can find probiotics in dairy foods, fermented foods and yogurt. New technology is putting probiotics in less traditional foods such as chocolate, cereal and other novel foods. When choosing a supplement, consider the potency, best species for your age and certain health conditions, production techniques, survivability and reliability. Foods, which offer an easy way to consume probiotics, are generally more accepted by the public than are supplements. Thanks to new innovations you can simply substitute a probiotic containing food for your regular food. On the other hand, supplements are more potent, convenient and the probiotics have better survivability than in foods. No matter which way you choose to get your probiotics, know that they will improve your health.

Multi-species probiotics are the best choice as they mimic your natural microflora and are supported in science as offering more health benefits than single species of probiotics. When targeting a specific illness, be sure to use the strain and potency used in the trials. Taking one million (10^8) CFUs is the minimum required in most studies to cause a health benefit. Regular use of probiotics is very important.

chapter
19
Common Probiotic Species

A MICROSCOPIC VIEW OF THIS CHAPTER

- Each species of probiotics has its own health benefits.
- Each strain of probiotics has its own characteristics.
- Diseases can be helped by more than one species.

■ ■ ■ ■ ■ ■ ■

There are many different types of probiotics. Probiotics come from a variety of bacterial and yeast families. A family of microbes has similar characteristics such as shape and the ideal locations for them to live in the body. Each strain has its own ability to affect your health. Researchers are working hard to learn more about each probiotic species. In fact, some researchers are trying to discover more microbes that offer you health benefits.

To date, there is no one "ultimate" probiotic species. Research commonly finds that a combination of a number of different probiotic species offers the best health benefits. Below is a detailed description of most of the probiotic species used in probiotic supplements and foods today. You will discover that some of them are well known to support health and fight some diseases.

BIFIDOBACTERIUM BREVE

B. breve is a gram-positive bacteria which can produce lactic acid. B. breve is found in the lower intestinal tract of infants and in some adults as well as in the adult vagina. This species' origin is from infant feces. Researchers have found *B. breve* to be capable of inhibiting *E. coli* and to be beneficial in people suffering from infectious diarrhea.

BIFIDOBACTERIUM BIFIDUM

B. bifidum is a dominant species in the mucus membrane that lines the large intestine and vaginal tract. *B. bifidum* has antimicrobial actions. It prevents the colonization of invading pathogenic bacteria by attaching to the intestinal wall, crowding out and taking nutrients from the bad microbes. *B. bifidum* is a lactic acid bacterium and as such it produces lactic acid and acetic acids. The production of these acids by *B. bifidum* lowers the pH of the intestinal environment, further inhibiting the growth of bad microbes. Research on Bifidobacteria has found that these probiotics enhance the assimilation of minerals such as iron, calcium, magnesium and zinc, all of which are essential for proper bone health.

BIFIDOBACTERIA INFANTIS

B. infantis is an important probiotic often found in the lower intestinal tract of humans. It has been shown to stimulate the production of immunomodulating agents such as cytokines. It positively influences the immune system. Researchers have also found *B. infantis* to have an antibacterial effect against pathogens such as Clostridia, Shigella and Salmonella.

BIFIDOBACTERIA LACTIS

B. lactis is a probiotic found in large numbers in the large intestine. Resistant to stomach acid and bile salts, this probiotic is a good candidate for effectively reaching the intestines after oral consumption. Research has found that *B. lactis* offers beneficial effects in patients with eczema. *B. lactis* appears to increase T-lymphocytes and natural killer cells and thus beneficially enhances the immune system.

BIFIDOBACTERIUM LONGUM

B. longum is a lactic acid bacteria that can excrete both lactic acid and acetic acid into the environment. Its resistance to acidic pH and bilary salts makes it a great candidate for oral supplementation. In addition, this probiotic is of human origin, which means it is likely to colonize and set up camp in the human intestinal tract to offer maximum health benefits. Known to have antimicrobial effects, it has been found in clinical studies to be effective against diarrhea and other infectious diseases. *B. longum* can stimulate the immune system and appears to offer some cancer prevention. *B. longum* is prominent in healthy children, and has been found to be beneficial against some childhood diseases. In addition, in clinical studies *B. longum* has been found to reduce the frequency of gastrointestinal disorders such as diarrhea and nausea during antibiotic use.

ENTEROCOCCUS FAECIUM

Enterococcus is a gram-positive bacterium with a spherical to ovoid shape. It is found in the intestinal microflora of humans and animals. Clinical research has used the strain SF68 successfully for the management of diarheal illness, particularly in cases where pathogenic microbes, such as Rotavirus, invade the bowel. One study found that *E. faecium* was more effective than *L. acidophilus* in shortening the duration of diarrheal episodes. It has a strong activity against a variety of pathogenic organisms. *E. faecium* only transiently colonizes the gastrointestinal tract. It is safe and has been extensively researched by the World Health Organization. Studies show it may also lower LDL cholesterol.

LACTOBACILLUS ACIDOPHILUS

L. acidophilus is a lactic acid bacterium with the ability to produce hydrogen peroxide. This may be one of the reasons it is effective in inhibiting pathogenic microorganisms from inhabiting and growing in the body. *L. acidophilus* produces natural antibacterials called *lactocidin* and *acidophilin*. These enhance resistance to pathogens. It is known to have an effective antimicrobial effect against *Staphylococcus aureus*, Salmonella, *E. coli* Rotavirus and *Candida albicans*. It is naturally found in human and animals, and thus colonizes well in the human digestive tract. *L. acidophilus* is one of the most well-known probiotics due to its natural presence in yogurt. It takes up residence in the small intestine, vagina, urethra and cervix. It aids in the production of niacin, folic acid and pyridoxine, three B vitamins. It may lower serum cholesterol. *L. acidophilus* has been found in clinical studies to be effective against antibiotic-associated diarrhea and appears to offer health benefits to people suffering from atopic disease, including dermatitis. Resistant to stomach acid and bile salts, this probiotic is a good candidate for effectively reaching the intestines after oral consumption.

LACTOBACILLUS BREVIS

L. brevis is a lactic acid bacterium that appears to be important to the synthesis of vitamins D and K. Research has shown that it may also be effective against *H. pylori* infections.

LACTOBACILLUS BULGARICUS

L. bulgaricus is a lactic acid–producing bacteria of dairy origin. It is resistant to acidic pH and bilary salts. It has antimicrobial effects and appears to offer beneficial effects in those suffering from diarrhea and infectious diseases. *L. bulgaricus* produces lactase, which can benefit those with lactose intolerance. It may offer some cancer prevention. *L. bulgaricus* has been used in clinical studies involving children with good success. Considered a transient microorganism, *L. bulgaricus* does not implant in the intestinal tract, but it still provides an important protective/beneficial role. Used in the commercial fermentation of yogurt, *L. bulgaricus* is a commonly consumed probiotic. Studies indicate that certain strains of *L. bulgaricus* stimulate production of interferon and tumor necrosis factor, thus stimulating and enhancing the immune system. In addition, *L. bulgaricus* helps to correct either constipation or diarrhea by significantly influencing the peristaltic action (rippling motion of muscles in the digestive tract) of the gastrointestinal tract.

LACTOBACILLUS CASEI

L. casei is a lactic acid–producing bacterium of human origin. It is closely related to *L. rhamnosus* and *L. acidophilus* and has some of the same immuno-modulating effects as other *Lactobacilli* species. It has been found in research studies to offer health benefits to those suffering from diarrhea and infectious disease. This may be due to its ability to produce bacteriocins, which are compounds that inhibit the growth of pathogenic bacteria in the small intestine. *L. casei* may offer some preventative effects against cancer. *L. casei* is beneficial to those who are lactose intolerant, as it aids in the digestion of lactose. *L. casei* is sometimes referred to as *L. casei* subspecies *paracasei*, and *L. casei* subspecies *rhamnosus*.

LACTOBACILLUS HELVETICUS

L. helveticus is a probiotic of dairy origin. It is a lactic acid bacteria that has antimicrobial effects. Research suggests that *L. helveticus* offers some preventative effects against cancer. Clinical research indicates that *L. helveticus* may be beneficial to those with hypertension.

LACTOCOCCUS LACTIS

A lactic acid bacteria, *L. lactis* is of dairy origin. Research has found *L. lactis* has antimicrobial effects and is capable of inhibiting the growth of bad microbes. It may offer some preventative effects against cancer. *L. lactis* is also known to help fight oral disease and diseases of the urogenital and vaginal tracts.

LACTOBACILLUS PLANTARUM

One of the probiotics of vegetal origin, this lactic acid–producing bacteria has a wide array of health benefits. It has immune-stimulating effects in the human body. *L. plantarum* secretes lactolin, a natural antibacterial and is known to have the ability to synthesize the amino acid lysine, which, in high quantities, has an anti-viral effect against some viruses such as the herpes virus which causes cold sores. *L. plantarum* can eradicate pathogens such as *S. aureus* in laboratory tests. Research suggests that *L. plantarum* offers health effects that may benefit people with allergies, arthritis, high cholesterol, infectious diseases and irritable bowel syndrome. *L. plantarum* may also offer preventative effects against cancer. In a clinical trial, *L. plantarum* reduced flatulence in patients with irritable bowel syndrome.

LACTOBACILLUS REUTERI

L. reuteri is one of the most studied species as it offers two unique features. *L. reuteri* produces reuterin, an antimicrobial substance that has been found to be effective against many pathogenic microbes including Rotavirus. *L. reuteri* is a gram-positive, lactic acid bacteria that was originally isolated from human breast milk and is also found in most mammals' intestines. Effective in infants and children suffering from Rotavirus infections, *L. reuteri* can reduce the severity and duration of diarrhea. It is also effective against antibiotic-associated diarrhea and traveler's diarrhea. It may also be effective against diarrhea caused by *Clostridium difficile*. Its antimicrobial actions also appear to eradicate *Helicobacter pylori*, the bacteria associated with ulcer formation in the stomach. *L. reuteri* has beneficial effects on the immune system and appears to be useful in those with atopic diseases. In North America, this species is only available in supplements offered by Nature's Way.

LACTOBACILLUS RHAMNOSUS

Originally placed under *L. casei*, *L. rhamnosus* is thought to share many of the immune-modulating effects of *L. casei*. Resistant to stomach acid and bile salts, this probiotic is a good candidate for effectively reaching the intestines after oral consumption. A lactic acid producer, *L. rhamnosus* is found in the small intestine and vaginal tract. As such, it is not surprising that it is effective in inhibiting those bacteria involved in vaginal and urinary tract infections. *L. rhamnosus* is very prolific in growth. It grows rapidly in milk and is found in many fermented dairy products. Its growth ability allows it to quickly establish in the human intestinal tract. It has a high tolerance to bile salts and adheres to the intestinal mucosa, protecting against invading microbes. *L. rhamnosus* has antimicrobial activity and is effective in people suffering from diarrhea. Research suggests it may also down-regulate hypersensitivity and thus help in those suffering from intestinal inflammation, atopic diseases, food allergies and more. *L. rhamnosus* has been found to have significant benefits in the nutrition and well-being of infants and in the elderly. In the large intestine, *L. rhamnosus* inhibits the growth of Streptococci and Clostridia and creates conditions favorable to Bifidobacteria growth.

LACTOBACILLUS RHAMNOSUS GG

One particular strain of *L. rhamnosus* has been the subject of extensive research. *Lactobacillus* GG, named after the surnames of its discoverers Dr. Sherwood Gorbach and Dr. Barry Golden, was discovered in 1985. *Lactobacillus* GG is resistant to stomach acid and bile, which enables it to survive the passage from the mouth to the small intestines with minimal loss to numbers. In the small intestines, *Lactobacillus* GG can adhere to the intestinal mucosa and proliferate. It's sold in over 30 countries in Asia, Europe and Latin America in products such as yogurt, milk drinks, cheese, juices and capsules. In North America, it's sold under the name Culturelle. *Lactobacillus* GG has been researched in many clinical trials and has been found to offer many health benefits for a variety of diseases.

LACTOBACILLUS SALIVARIUS

L. salivarius helps normalize the intestinal flora in those suffering from chronic bowel conditions such as irritable bowel syndrome. It is a lactic acid bacteria. *L. salivarius* may be an effective inhibitor of the bacteria *H. pylori*, a bacteria associated with the formation of ulcers in the stomach. *L. salivarius* also appears to reduce flatulence.

PROPIONIBACTERIA

Species of *Propionibacteria* can be found all over the body. *Propionibacteria* are generally nonpathogenic; however, they can cause a number of infections, including the common skin disease acne vulgaris, which is caused by *P. acnes*. *P. freudenreichii* is used in Swiss cheese manufacturing to produce its flavor and characteristic holes. *P. freudenreichii* appears to offer health benefits to the host. In a clinical trial, *P. freudenreichii* was able to increase defecation frequency in elderly humans. It may also alleviate some symptoms of irritable bowel syndrome in combination with *L. rhamnosus* and *B. breve*.

SACCHAROMYCES BOULARDII

S. boulardii is a yeast and a probiotic. It is also known as *Saccharomyces cerevisiae*. Interestingly, it was first isolated from lychee and mangosteen fruit in 1923. Clinical trials have shown it is effective at improving health in those with diarrhea associated with antibiotic use, as well as traveler's diarrhea. It may help with diarrhea caused by *C. difficile*. Research has shown that *S. boulardii* may be beneficial for those suffering from irritable bowel disease, ulcerative colitis and Crohn's disease.

STREPTOCOCCUS THERMOPHILUS

S. thermophilus is found in dairy products such as yogurt. Resistant to stomach acid and bile salts, this probiotic is a good candidate for effectively reaching the intestines after oral consumption. It is efficient in breaking down lactose by producing the enzyme lactase, which is deficient in those with lactose intolerance. *S. thermophilus* is immune stimulating. It can stimulate the production of cytokine, a chemical used by the immune system to communicate and organize attacks against threatening bacteria and viruses *S. thermophilus* has been found in research to have antimicrobial effects, to lower cholesterol and to offer some benefits to those suffering from infectious diseases, diarrhea, children's diseases and diseases of the skin, urogenital tract and vagina.

Appendices

APPENDIX 3-1

Human Disease Conditions and the Probiotics Known to Promote
Health in These Conditions

Condition	Probiotic Therapy	Results
Diarrhea (infectious)	B. bifidum	Less frequent stools
Diarrhea (antibiotic-associated)	B. lactis S. thermophilus	Less frequent stools Decreases incidence
Candida	L. acidophilus	Weakens the infection
Chlamydia	E. faecium	Reduces infection
C. rodentium	L. acidophilus L. rhamnosus	Reduces cell growth in colon
Giardia	E. faecium	Reduces infection
Helicobacter pylori	L. acidophilus L. rhamnosus L. gasseri L. reuteri	Reduces inflammation Decreases H. pylori growth
Salmonella	B. longum S. cerevisiae L. reuteri	Reduces infection
C. difficile	S. cerevisiae	Reduces rate of death in patients

APPENDIX 3-2

Bifidobacteria Species Known to Inhibit Infection of Pathogens
That Cause Disease in Humans

Bifidobacteria Species	Pathogen Inhibited	Reference
B. longum	Salmonella typhimurium	Silva et al. 1999
B. breve	E. coli	Asahara et al. 2004
B. pseudocatenulatum	E. coli	Gagnon et al. 2004
Bifidobacterium	Listeria monocytogenes	Toure et al. 2003
	Campylobacter jejuni	Fooks and Gibson 2003
	Bacteroides vulgatus	Shiba et al. 2003

APPENDIX 4-1

Common Commercially Used Probiotic Species

Lactobacillus
L. acidophilus
L. delbrueckii ssp bulgaricus
L. fermentum
L. gasseri
L. johnsonii
L. lactis
L. paracasei
L. plantarum
L. reuteri
L. rhamnosus GG (L. casei)
L. salivarius
Bifidobacterium
B. adolescentis
B. animalis
B. bifidum

B. breve
B. catenulatum
B. infantis
B. lactis
B. longum
B. regularis (B. animalis)
Enterococcus
E. faecium
E. faecalis
Streptococcus
S. thermophilus
Other
Saccharomyces boulardii (S. cerevisiae)
Oxalobacter formigenes
Bacillus cereus
Bacillus subtilis
Bacillus coagulans
Escherichia coli
Streptococcus thermophilus
Propionibacterium freudenrechii

APPENDIX 4-2

Bifidobacterium species in the intestine of infants and adults (according to Lerche and Reuter, 1961; Reuter, 1963, 1971; Mitsuoka, 1969, 1982).

Bifidobacteria	Strain (biotype)	Present in Infants	Present in Adults
B. bifidum	a	*	+
	b	+	*
B. adolescentis	a	+	+
	b		+

continued

Bifidobacteria	Strain (biotype)	Present in Infants	Present in Adults
	c	*	+
	d		(+)
B. longum	a	*	+
	b	+	*
B. infantis	c	+	
	d	+	
B. breve	a	(+)	*
	b	*	
	c	*	

Frequency:
+ frequently
(+) moderately
* occasionally

Source: Lerche and Reuter, 1961; Reuter, 1963, 1971; Mitsuoka, 1969, 1982.

APPENDIX 4-3

Some of the Human Disease Conditions Known to Benefit from Oral Administration of Certain Probiotic Species.

Disease Condition	Probiotic Therapy	Results
Asthma	L. rhamnosus	Decreased incidence
Atopic dermatitis	B. lactis	Reduced symptoms
	L. casei	
	L. fermentum	
	L. reuteri	
	L. rhamnosus	
Bladder cancer	L. casei Shirota	Reduced recurrence
Candida	L. acidophilus	Reduced infection
	L. crispatus	
	L. fermentum	
	L. jensenii	
	L. rhamnosus	
C. difficile	S. cerevisiae	Reduced risk of death

Disease Condition	Probiotic Therapy	Results
Colic	*L. reuteri*	Reduced crying time
Colon cancer	*B. animalis*	Reduced risk
	B. breve	
	B. lactis	
	B. longum	
	L. rhamnosus	
Common Cold	*B. bifidum*	Reduced incidence
	B. longum	
	L. gasseri	
Diarrhea (infectious)	*B. bifidum*	Less frequent stools
	B. breve	
	B. lactis	
	*L. casei**	
	L. reuteri	
	L. rhamnosus	
	S. thermophilus	
Diarrhea	*B. bifidum*	Less frequent stools
(antibiotic-associated)	*B. lactis*	Decreased incidence
	B. longum	of diarrhea
	E. faecium	
	L. acidophilus	
	L. bulgaricus	
	S. boulardii	
	S. thermophilus	
E. coli	*L. acidophilus*	Reduced infection
	L. rhamnosus	
Giardia	*E. faecium*	Reduced infection
Helicobacter pylori	*L. acidophilus*	Decreased *H. pylori* or
	L. brevis	inhibited growth
	*L. casei**	
	L. gasseri	
	L. johnsonii La1	

continued

Disease Condition	Probiotic Therapy	Results
	L. reuteri	
	L. rhamnosus	
	L. salivarius	
	S. boulardii	
High Cholesterol	*B. longum*	Improved cholesterol
	E. faecium	levels
	L. acidophilus	
Irritable Bowel Disease	*B. breve*	Reduced bowel
(Crohn's disease)	*B. infantis*	movements
	B. longum	
	L. acidophilus	
	L. bulgaricus	
	L. casei*	
	L. plantarum	
	L. salivarus	
	S. thermophilus	
	S. boulardii	
	VSL#3	
Irritable Bowel Disease	*L. casei**	Clinical remission/
(Ulcerative colitis)	*S. boulardii*	Reduced inflammation
	S. thermophilus	and infection
	VSL#3	
Irritable Bowel	*B. infantis*	Less bloating/
Syndrome (IBS)	*B. lactis*	Decreased pain
	L. acidophilus	
	L. paracasei	
	L. plantarum	
	L. rhamnosus	
	L. salivarius	
	VSL#3	
Lactose intolerance	*B. animalis*	Assist lactose digestion
	B. longum	

Disease Condition	Probiotic Therapy	Results
	L. acidophilus	
	L. bulgaricus	
	S. thermophilus	
Liver cancer	L. rhamnosus	Reduced carcinogens
	P. freudenreichii	
Oral health (dental carries)	L. casei*	Improved health
	L. bulgaricus	Reduced development
	L. lactis	of dental carries
	L. paracasei	
	L. rhamnosus	
	S. thermophilus	
Pouchitis	L. casei*	
	S. thermophilus	
	VSL#3	
Salmonella	B. longum	Reduced infection
	L. reuteri	
	S. cerevisiae	
Traveler's Diarrhea	L. casei*	Reduced incidences
	S. boulardii	
Ulcers	L. casei	Speeds healing time
Urinary Tract Infection (UTI)	L. casei Shirota	Prevented infection
	L. crispatus	
	L. fermentum	
	L. reuteri	
	L. rhamnosus	
Vaginosis	L. acidophilus	Prevented infection
	L. crispatus	
	L. delbrueckii	
	L. fermentum	
	L. paracasei	
	L. rhamnosus	

continued

Disease Condition	Probiotic Therapy	Results
Yeast Infections	*L. acidophilus* *L. fermentum* *L. rhamnosus*	Reduced infection

L. rhamnosus GG is commonly called *L. casei*

APPENDIX 6-1

Bad Microbes That Can Cause Diarrhea

Diarrhea-Causing Microbes	Examples
Bacteria	Campylobacter, Salmonella, Shigella, *Escherichia coli*
Viral	Rotavirus, Norwalk, Cytomegalovirus, Hepatitis
Parasite	*Giardia lambia, Entamoeba histolytica,* Cryptosporidium
Food Intolerance	Unable to digest food components, e.g., lactose
Reaction to Medicine	Antibiotics, some blood pressure and cancer medications
Intestinal Disease	Colitis, Crohn's disease, Celiac disease
Functional Bowel Disorders	Irritable bowel syndrome
Vitamin C	Over dosage of vitamin C can cause diarrhea

APPENDIX 6-2

Reported Effects of Probiotic Species on Diarrhea in Children and Infants

Probiotic Strain	Reported Clinical Effect	Age	Reference
B. bifidum	Reduces incidence of Rotavirus infection	Infants	Saavedra et al. 1994

Probiotic Strain	Reported Clinical Effect	Age	Reference
S. thermophilus	Reduces incidence of Rotavirus infection	Infants	Saavedra et al. 1994
B. breve	Inhibits ability of Rotavirus to infect host	Infants and Children	Bae et al. 2002
B. lactis	Positively treats acute diarrhea	Children	Chouraqui et al. 2004
L. reuteri *(+ L. rhamnosus)*	Shortens duration of acute diarrhea	Daycare children	Rosenfeldt et al. 2002
L. reuteri *(+ L. rhamnosus)*	Reduces hospitalization rate and diarrhea in children	Hospitalized children	Rosenfeldt et al. 2002
L. rhamnosus *(+ L. reuteri)*	Shortens duration of acute diarrhea	Daycare children	Rosenfeldt et al. 2002
L. rhamnosus *(+ L. reuteri)*	Reduces hospitalization rate and diarrhea in children	Hospitalized children	Rosenfeldt et al. 2002
L. reuteri	Reduces duration of watery diarrhea	Children (6 – 36 months)	Shornikova et al. 1997
Bifidobacteria	Protects against symptomatic Rotavirus infection	Children (6 – 36 months)	Phuapradit et al. 1999
S. thermophilus *(+ B. bifidum)*	Reduces incidence of acute diarrhea	Infants (5 – 24 months)	Tomsen 2006
L. casei	Reduces incidence of acute diarrhea in children	Infants (6 – 24 months)	Pedone et al. 2000

APPENDIX 12-1

Food Sources of Calcium

Food Item	Portion	Calcium (mg)
Almonds	3 oz	210
Broccoli (cooked)	2 stalks	250

continued

Food Item	Portion	Calcium (mg)
Collard greens (cooked)	6 oz	225
Dried apricots	3 oz	80
Egg yolk	1	25
Fortified margarine	2 tsp	51
Fortified orange juice	1/2 cup	45
Fortified rice or soy beverage	1 cup	80
Herring or trout, cooked	75 g	156
Mackerel, cooked	75 g	80
Milk	1 cup	100
Salmon, Atlantic, cooked	75 g	225
Salmon, canned or cooked*	75 g	608
Sardines, Atlantic, canned	75 g	70
Sardines, Pacific, canned	75 g	360
Sunflower seeds	2 oz	80
Tuna, canned, light or white	75 g	41
Tuna, canned, yellow fin (albacore, ahi)	75 g	105
Yogurt	6 oz	300

*includes Chinook, Coho, Humpback (pink), Sockeye

APPENDIX 18-1

Origins of Some Probiotic Species

Human Origins
B. adolescentis – adult feces
B. angulatum – adult feces
B. bifidum – child and adult feces, vagina
B. breve – child feces, vagina
B. catenulatum – child and adult feces, vagina
B. denticolens – buccal cavity
B. dentium – buccal cavity, adult feces
B. gallicum – adult feces
B. infantis – child feces, vagina

B. inopinatum – buccal cavity
B. longum – child and adult feces and vagina
B. pseudocatenulatum – child feces
Environmental and Food Origins
B. lactis – fermented milk
B. minimum – sewage
B. subtile – sewage
B. thermacidophilum – anaerobic digester
Animal Origins
B. animalis – rat, chicken, rabbit and calf feces
B. asteroides – bees
B. boum – rumen, piglet feces
B. choerinum –piglet feces
B. coryneforme – bees
B. cuniculi – rabbit feces
B. gallinarum – chicken feces
B. indicum – bees
B. magnum – rabbit feces
B. merycicuum – rumen
B. pseudolongum – piglet, chicken, calf, rat feces
B. pullorum – chicken feces
B. ruminantium – rumen
B. saeculare – rabbit feces
B. suis – piglet feces
B. thermophilum – piglet, chicken and calf feces

APPENDIX 18-2

Some Commercial Food Products with Added Probiotics

Strain(s)	Commercial Products
L. casei DN114001 (L. casei Defensis ™)	DanActive® fermented milk
B. lactis Bb-12	Good Start Natural Cultures® infant formula

continued

Strain(s)	Commercial Products
L. casei Shirota, *B. breve* strain Yakult	Yakult®
L. acidophilus, *L. casei* (CL 1285)	Bio-K+®
B. animalis DN173 010 (Bifidis regularis™)	Danone Activia® yogurt
L. johnsonii Lj-1 (same as NCC533 and formerly *L. acidophilus* La-1)	LC1® Go!
L. reuteri SD2112	Stonyfield Farms yogurts
L. rhamnosus GG (LGG)	Dannon Danimals®
Lactobacillus bulgaricus, *Streptococcus thermophilus*, *Lactobacillus casei*	Horizon® Organic Yogurts
Lactobacillus acidophilus LA5, *Bifidobacterium lactis* BB12	Yoplait Yoptimal Immun+
L. casei Defensive, *L. casei* Immunitass	Danone Actimel
L. casei	Kashi Vive Cereal
L. acidophilus (LAFTI ®L10), *L. casei* (LAFTI® L26), *B. lactis* (LAFTI® B94)	Attune Snack Bars
L. rhamnosus, *B. lactis*	Kraft LiveActive

Glossary

acidic Acid forming; acid—having a pH of less than 7.

acute Short term.

alkaline Relating to, containing or having the properties of an alkali or alkali metal; basic or having a pH of more than 7.

anaphylactic shock A serious, often life-threatening allergic reaction that is characterized by low blood pressure, shock and difficulty breathing.

angiogenesis The process of developing new blood vessels.

animal model An animal sufficiently like humans in its anatomy, physiology or response to a pathogen to be used in medical research in order to obtain results that can be extrapolated to human medicine.

antibacterial Destructive to or inhibiting the growth of bacteria.

antibody A protein with a specific structure designed for an antigen; tags an antigen to help the immune system identify and destroy it; can be produced due to first exposure or can be made from memory of a previous exposure.

antibiotic A substance produced by or a semisynthetic substance derived from a microorganism and, in dilute solution, able to inhibit or kill another microorganism.

antigen A molecule whose shape triggers the production of antibodies (immunoglobulins) that will bind to the antigen. A foreign substance capable of triggering an immune response in an organism.

antimicrobial Destroying or inhibiting the growth of microorganisms, especially pathogenic microorganisms.

apoptosis A form of cell death in which a programmed sequence of events leads to the elimination of cells without releasing harmful substances into the surrounding area.

atopic disease Allergic diseases such as asthma and eczema produced upon exposure, especially by inhalation, to an environmental antigen.

bacteria Any of the unicellular prokaryotic microorganisms of the class *Schizomycetes*, which vary in terms of morphology, oxygen and nutritional requirements, and motility; may be free-living, saprophytic, or pathogenic in plants or animals.

bacteriocins Proteins produced by bacteria that are toxic to other species.

Bifidobacteria Rod-shaped, gram-positive, non-acid-fast, non-spore-forming, non-motile bacterium that is a genus of the family *Actinomycetaceae*. It inhabits the intestines and feces of humans as well as the human vagina.

bifidogenic A product that stimulates Bifidobacteria growth or activity.

carcinogen A substance that promotes the development of cancer.

carcinogenic Any substance, radionuclide or radiation that is an agent directly involved in the promotion of cancer or in the facilitation of its propagation. This may be due to genomic instability or to the disruption of cellular metabolic processes.

CFU Colony-forming units; a measurement used to count bacteria/microbes. Scientists call any microbes that can be counted a colony.

colonization The formation of compact population groups of the same type of microorganism; colonies that develop when a bacterial cell begins reproducing.

colon The large intestine; the last section of the intestinal tract; responsible for forming, storing and excreting waste matter.

cytokine Small proteins produced by cells that have an effect on cell-to-cell interaction, communication and behavior of cells.

dermatitis Inflammation of the skin.

duodenum The first or proximal portion of the small intestine, extending from the pylorus to the jejunum, so called because it is about 12 finger-lengths long.

dysbiosis The state of a disordered microbial ecology that causes disease.

enteric General term for the intestines.

epithelial Any animal tissue that covers a surface, or lines a cavity or the like, and that, in addition, performs any of various secretory, transporting or regulatory functions.

eradicate To destroy utterly.

etiology Cause or underlying reason for disease development.

gastroenteritis Inflammation of the stomach and intestines.

genera Plural of genus.

genus The taxonomic classification used as a prefix to a species, such as the genus *homo* sapiens.

humoral immunity The component of the immune system involving antibodies that are secreted by B cells and circulate as soluble proteins in blood plasma and lymph.

hygiene hypothesis Suggested by David Strachan in 1989 that the increasing rates of allergy-based diseases in developed countries is due to infants' decreased exposure to microbes and allergens due to increased hygiene standards.

fermentation An energy-yielding process whereby organic molecules serve as both electron donors and electron accepters.

flagella A hair-like projection on some bacteria cells that provides movement for the cell.

hypocholesterolemic To cause a decrease in blood cholesterol levels.

ileum The last portion of the small intestine; found between the duodenum and the colon; hosts enzyme-controlled actions that break down food.

immunological Of or relating to immunology.

jejunum The portion of the small intestine that extends from the duodenum to the ileum.

lactic acid bacteria Bacteria that produce lactic acid as a metabolic waste product and secrete it into their environment.

Lactobacilli Milk bacteria; normally found in the mouth, intestinal tract and vagina.

leaky gut syndrome A condition in which fluids, antigens and microbes can breach the intestinal lining and enter the circulatory system.

lumen The inner open space or cavity of a tubular organ; as of a blood vessel or an intestine.

lymphocyte White blood cells; more specifically the cellular mediators of immunity that constitute 20% to 30% of the white blood cells in normal human blood.

lymphoid tissue Area of cells that is rich in white blood cells such as macrophages; includes the lymph nodes, spleen, tonsils and adenoids, and the thymus.

membrane A thin layer of phospholipids (fat-like molecules) that line the outside of cells and organelles (compartments found within a cell).

microbe Another term for microorganisms, including bacteria, viruses, yeasts, fungi, protozoa and algae.

microbial Of, relating to, caused by, or being microbes.

microflora The bacteria and fungi that inhabit an area.

microorganism A microscopic organism; those of medical interest include bacteria, viruses, algae, fungi and protozoa. An organism of microscopic size; not visible to the human eye.

necrotisis Death of living tissue.

pancreas An organ lying below and behind the stomach that secretes bile salts containing cholesterol and enzymes to help with the digestion of food. It secretes the hormones insulin and glucagon (both regulate blood sugar).

pathogen Any disease-producing microorganism.

pathogenic Capable of causing disease.

phenotype The outward, physical manifestation of an organism.

placebo Treatment given in a blinded study that has no effect on the outcome of the subjects; commonly referred to as the "nothing treatment" or the "sugar-pill."

prebiotic Nondigestible food ingredients that may beneficially affect the host by selectively stimulating the growth and or metabolic activity of one or a limited number of bacteria in the colon and thus improve health.

probiotic Live microorganisms which, when administered in adequate amounts, confer a health benefit on the host.

omeprazole A proton pump-inhibitor drug commonly used to treat gastric reflux.

rumen The first of four stomachs in ruminant animals, such as cattle or deer.

secondhand smoke A combination of the smoke that is released from the end of a burning cigarette and the smoke exhaled from the lungs of smokers.

short chain fatty acids A small fat found in the human body that contains less than eight carbons.

species A taxonomic category subordinate to a genus (or subgenus) and superior to a subspecies or variety, composed of individual organisms possessing common characteristics distinguishing them from other categories of individual organisms of the same taxonomic level.

Staph: *Staphylococcus aureus*, a bacteria that can become resistant to antibiotic treatments.

strain A subset of a bacterial species differing from other bacteria of the same species by some minor, but identifiable, difference. A strain is a population of organisms that descends from a single organism or pure culture isolate. Strains within a species may differ slightly from one another in many ways. An example is *B. lactis* BB12.

Streptococci A group of spherical, gram-positive bacteria. In addition to strep throat, Streptococcus species are responsible for many cases of meningitis, bacterial pneumonia, endocarditis, erysipelas and necrotizing fasciitis. Many Streptococcal species are non-pathogenic. Streptococci are also part of the normal flora of the mouth, skin, intestine and upper respiratory tract of humans.

subspecies A taxonomic group that is a division of a species.

symbiotic A close, long relationship between two different organisms which may be beneficial.

synbiotic Nutritional supplements containing probiotics and prebiotics.

synergistically Relating to synergy; acting together; enhancing the effect of another force or agent.

taxinomical Relating to taxonomy; the theories and techniques of naming, describing and classifying organisms.

transient Short-lived; passing; not permanent.

translocation The movemet of particles in the intestinal tract across the intestinal lining and into the bloodstream.

toxicology The study of the nature, effects and detection of poisons and the treatment of poisoning.

toxicological Of or relating to toxicology.

urogenital Anatomical reference pertaining to the urinary and genital apparatus.

villi Of-the-minute, worm-like processes on certain membranes, especially on the mucous membrane of the small intestine, that help the body to absorb nutrients.

virus shedding A process by which viruses are expelled from the body; a form of disease transmission.

VSL#3 A group of probiotic strains used in combination in clinical trials: *L. casei, L. plantarum, L. acidophilus, L. bulgaricus, B. longum, B. breve, B. infantis* and *S. thermophilus*.

visceral sensory system Referring to the internal organs of the body; a neurological structure that supports communication between the internal organs and the brain.

References

CHAPTER 1

Bergonzelli, G.E., et al. Probiotics as a treatment strategy for gastrointestinal diseases? *Digestion,* 2005; 72:57–68.

Food and Agriculture Organization (FAO) of the United Nations and World Health Organization (WHO). *Guidelines for the Evaluation of Probiotics in Food.* Report of a Joint FAO/WHO Working Group on Drafting Guidelines for the Evaluation of Probiotics in Food. Accessed on December 7, 2006.

Gibson, G.R. and Roberfroid, M.B. Dietary modulation of the human colonic microbiota: introducing the concept of prebiotics. *Journal of Nutrition,* 1995; 125:1401–1412.

Marteau, P., Seksik, P., and R. Jian. Probiotics and intestinal health effects: a clinical perspective. *British Journal of Nutrition,* 2002; 88(1): S51–57.

Ouwehand, A. and S. Vesterlund. Health aspects of probiotics. *The Investigational Drugs Journal,* 2003; 6(6):573–580.

What Canadians should know about Gastro-Intestinal disease. Press Release. *Canadian Association of Gastroenterology,* September 2005.

CHAPTER 2

Leahy, S.C. et al. Getting better with *bifidobacteria. Journal of Applied Microbiology* 2005; 98:1303–1315.

Metchnikoff, Elie. *Encyclopaedia Britannica 2007*. Encyclopaedia Britannica Online. May 2007. http://www.britannica.com/eb/article-9052307.

Schrezenmeir, Jürgen and de Vrese, Michael. Probiotics, prebiotics, and synbiotics—approaching a definition. *American Journal of Clinical Nutrition*, 2001; 73(2):361S–364S.

CHAPTER 3

Ashara, T., et al. Probiotic bifidobacteria protect mice from lethal infection with shiga toxin-producing Escherichia coli 0157:H7. *Infection and Immunity*, 2000; 72:2240–2247.

Axelsson, L., et al. Production of a broad spectrum antimicrobial substance by *Lactobacillus reuteri*. *Microbial Ecology Health Disease*, 1989; 2:2131–2136.

Banasaz, M., et al. Increased enterocyte production in gnotobiotic rats mono-associated with *Lactobacillus rhamnosus*. *Environmental Microbioogy*, 2002 June; 68(6):3031–3034.

Centers for Disease Control and Prevention, Coordinating Center for Infectious Diseases/Division of Bacterial and Mycotic Diseases November 4, 2006.

Dai, D. and Walker, W. A. Protective nutrients and bacterial colonization in the immature human gut. *Advances in Pediatrics*, 1999; 46:353–382.

Falagas, M.E., et al. Probiotics for prevention of recurrent vulvovaginal candidiasis: a review. *Journal of Antimicrobial Chemotherapy*, 2006; 58(2):266–72.

Fooks, L.J. and Gibson, G. R. Mixed culture fermentation studies on the effect of synbiotics on the human intestinal pathogens *Campylobacter jejuni* and *Escherichia coli*. *Anaerobe*, 2003; 9:231–242.

Fooks, L.J. and Gibson, G. R. Probiotics as modulators of the gut flora. *British Journal of Nutrition*, 2002; 88(S1); S39–S49.

Gagnon, M., et al. In vitro inhibition of Escherichia coli 0157:H7 by *bifidobacterial* strains of human origin. *International Journal of Food Microbiology*, 2004; 92:69–78.

Guandalini, S.L., et al. *Lactobacillus* GG administered in oral rehydration solution to children with acute diarrhea: a multicenter

European trial. *Journal of Pediatric Gastroenterology and Nutrition*, 2000, 30:54–60.

Hatakka, K., et al. Probiotics reduce the prevalence of oral *candida* in the elderly—a randomized controlled trial. *Journal of Dental Research*, 2007; 86(2):125–130.

Isolauri, E., et al. Probiotics: effects on immunity. *American Journal of Clinical Nutrition*, 2001; 73(2):444S–450S.

Johnson-Henry, K.C., et al. Probiotics in models of GI bacterial infections. *Nutrafood*, 2005; 4(2/3):29–36.

Kaewsrichan, J., et al. Selection and identification of anaerobic *lactobacilli* producing inhibitory compounds against vaginal pathogens. *FEMS Immunological Medical Microbiology*, 2006; 48(1):75–83.

Lu, L. and Walker, W.A. Pathologic and physiologic interactions of bacteria with the gastrointestinal epithelium. *American Journal of Clinical Nutrition*, 2001; 73:1124S–1130.

Ma, D., et al. Live *Lactobacillus reuteri* is essential for the inhibitory effect on tumor necrosis factor alpha-induced interleukin-8 expression. *Infection and Immunity*, 2004; 72(9):5308–5314.

Rakoff-Nahoum, S., et al. Recognition of commensal microflora by toll-like receptors is required for intestinal homeostasis. *Cell*, 2004; 118:229–241.

Ruiz-Palacios, G., et al. Feeding of a probiotic for the prevention of community-acquired diarrhea in young Mexican children. *Pediatric Research*, 1996; 39:184.

Saggioro, A., et al. Helicobacter pylori eradication with *lactobacillus reuteri*. A double-blind, placebo-controlled study. *Digestive and Liver Disease*, 2005; 37(1):S88.

Sharif, S. Antibiotic replacement therapy for control of food-borne pathogens in poultry. Ontario Ministry of Agriculture, Food and Rural Affairs, June 2006.

Shiba, T., et al. The suppressive effect of bifidobacteria on Bacteroides vulgatas, a putatitve pathogenic microbe in inflammatory bowel disease. *Microbiology and Immunology*, 2003; 47:371–378.

Shornikova, A., et al. *Lactobacillus reuteri* as a therapeutic agent in acute diarrhea in young children. *Journal of Pediatric Gastroenterology and Nutrition*, 1997; 24:399–404.

Shornikova, A., et al. Bacteriotherapy with *Lactobacillus reuteri* in rotavirus gastroenteritis. *Pediatric Infectious Disease,* 1997; 16:1103–1107.

Silva, A.M., et al. Protective effect of bifidus milk on the experimental infection with Salmonella enteritidis subsp. typhimurium in conventional and gnotobiotic mice. *J Appl Microbiol,* 1999; 86:331–336.

Steer, T., et al. Perspectives on the role of the human gut microbiota and its modulation by pro and prebiotics. *Nutrition Research Reviews,* 2000; 13:229–254.

Strus, M., et al. The in vitro activity of vaginal *Lactobacillus* with probiotic properties against Candida. *Infectious Disease in Obstetrics and Gynecology,* 2005; 13(2):69–75.

Tomsen, M. Probiotics—enhancing health with beneficial bacteria. *Alternative and Complementary Therapy,* 2006 Feb.: 14–21.

Toure, R, et al. Production of antibacterial substances by *bifidobacterial* isolates from infant stool active against *Listeria monocytogenes*. *Journal of Applied Microbiology,* 2003; 95:1058–1069.

CHAPTER 4

Bentley, R. and R. Meganathan. Biosynthesis of vitamin K (menaquinone) in bacteria. *Bacteriological Reviews,* 1982; 46(3):241–280.

Bergonzelli, GE, et al. Probiotics as a treatment strategy for gastrointestinal diseases? *Digestion,* 2005; 72:57–68.

http://www.usprobiotics.org/basics/#Microbe%20Role%20in%20GI%20Tract.

Imase, K., et al. *Lactobacillus reuteri* tablets suppress *Helicobacter pylori* infection—a double-blind randomised placebo-controlled cross-over clinical study. *The Journal of the Japanese Association for Infectious Disease,* 2007; 81(4):387–93.

Leahy, S.C., et al. Getting better with *bifidobacteria. Journal of Applied Microbiology,* 2005; 98:1303–1315.

Lionetti, E., et al. *Lactobacillus reuteri* therapy to reduce side-effects during anti-*Helicobacter pylori* treatment in children: a randomized placebo controlled trial. *Alimentary Pharmacology and Therapeutics,* 2006 Nov 15; 24(10):1461–8.

Ouwehand, A. and Vesterlund, S. Health aspects of probiotics. *The Investigational Drugs Journal,* 2003; 6(6):573–580.

Rosenfeldt, V., et al. Effect of probiotic *Lactobacillus* strains on acute diarrhea in a cohort of non-hospitalized children attending day-care centres. *The Pediatric Infectious Disease Journal*, 2002; 21:417–9.

Tomsen, M. Probiotics—enhancing health with beneficial bacteria. *Alternative Complementary Therapy*, 2006: 14–21.

CHAPTER 5

Brighenti, F., et al. One month consumption of ready-to-eat breakfast cereal containing inulin markedly lowers serum lipids in normolipidemic men. 7th European Nutrition Conference. Vienna, Austria, May 24–28, 1995.

Coudray, C., et al. Effect of soluble or partly soluble dietary fibres supplementation on absorption and balance of calcium, magnesium, iron and zinc in healthy young men. *European Journal of Clinical Nutrition*, 1997; 51:375 380.

Fiordaliso, M., et al. Dietary oligofructose lowers triglycerides, phospholipids and cholesterol in serum and very low density liporpoteins in rats. *Lipids*, 1995; 30:163–167.

Gibson, G.R. and Roberfroid, M.B. Dietary modulation of the human colonic microbiota: introducing the concept of prebiotics. *Journal of Nutrition*, 1995; 125:1401–1412.

Manning, T.S. and Gibson, G.R. Prebiotics. *Best Practice and Research Clinical Gastroenterology*, 2004; 18:287–298.

Niness, K. Inulin and oligofructose: what are they? *Journal of Nutrition*, 1999; 129:1402S–1406S.

Taper, H., et al. Protective effect of dietary fructo-oligosaccharide in young rats against exocrine pancreas atrophy induced by high fructose and partial copper deficiency. *Food and Chemical Toxicology*, 1995; 33:631–639.

Van Loo, J., et al. On the presence of inulin and oligofructose as natural ingredients in the Western diet. *CRC Critical Reviews in Food Science and Nutrition*, 1995; 35:525–552.

CHAPTER 6

Bae, E.A., et al. Purification of rotavirus infection-inhibitory protein from *Bifidobacterium breve* K-110. *Journal of Microbiology Biotechnology*, 2002; 12:553–556.

Beaugerie, L. and Petit, J.C. Microbial-gut interactions in health and disease. Antibiotic associated diarrhea. *Best Practice and Research Clinical Gastroenterology*, 2004; 18:337–352.

Chouraqui, J.P., et al. Acidified milk formula supplemented with *Bifidobacterium lactis*: impact on infant diarrhea in residential care settings. *Journal of Pediatric Gastroenterology and Nutrition*, 2004; 38:288–292.

Colombel, J.F., et al. Yoghurt with *Bifidobacterium longum* reduces erythromycin-induced gastrointestinal effects. *Lancet*, 1987; 2:43.

Consumer Attitudes about Antibiotics and Antibiotic Resistance. Ipsos-Reid National Survey, January 29, 2002.

D'Souza, A.L., et al. Probiotics in prevention of antibiotic associated diarrhoea: meta-analysis. *British Medical Journal*, 2002; 324(7350):1361.

Isolauri, E. Probiotics for infectious diarrhea. *Gut*, 2003; 52: 435–437.

Marteau. P., et al. Probiotics and intestinal health effects: a clinical perspective. *British Journal of Nutrition*, 2002; 88(1):S51–S57.

Orrhage, K., et al. Effect of supplements of *Bifidobacterium longum* and *Lactobacillus acidophilus* on intestinal microbiota during administration of clindamycin. *Microbial Ecology in Health and Disease*, 1994; 7:17 25.

Ouwehand, A. and S. Vesterlund. Health aspects of probiotcs. *The Investigational Drugs Journal*, 2003; 6(6):573–580.

Pedone, C.A., et al. Multicentric study of the effect of milk fermented by *Lactobacillus casei* on the incidence of diarrhea. *International Journal of Clinical Practice*, 2000; 54(9):568–71.

Plummer, S., et al. *Clostridium difficile* pilot study: effect of probiotic supplementation on the incidence of C. difficile diarrhea. *International Microbiology*, 2004; 7:59–62.

Rosenfeldt, V., et al. Effect of probiotic *Lactobacillus* strains in young children hospitalized with acute diarrhea. *The Pediatric Infectious Disease Journal*, 2002; 21:411–16.

Saavedra, J.M., et al. Feeding of *Bifidobacterium bifidum* and *Streptococcus thermophilus* to infants in hospital for prevention of diarrhea and shedding of rotavirus. *Lancet*, 1994; 344:1046–1049.

Shornikova, A.V., et al. Bacteriotherapy with *Lactobacillus reuteri* in rotavirus gastroenteritis. *The Pediatric Infectious Disease Journal*, 1997; 16:1103–1107.

CHAPTER 7

Bennet, R. and Nord, C.E. The human intestinal microflora during the first year of life. Department of Paediatrics, St. Görans Hospital, S–112 81 Stockholm, Sweden, and Department of Microbiology, Huddinge University Hospital, Karolinska Institute, S–141 86 Huddinge, Sweden.

Marteau, P., et al. Probiotics and intestinal health effects: a clinical perspective. *British Journal of Nutrition*, 2002; 88(1):S51–S57.

Saavedra, J.M. Feeding of *Bifidobacterium bifidum* and *Streptococcus thermophilus* to infants in hospital for prevention of diarrhoea and shedding of rotavirus. *Lancet*, 1994; 344(8929):1046–1049.

Saavedra, J.M., et al. Long-term consumption of infant formulas containing live probiotic bacteria: tolerance and safety. *American Journal of Clinical Nutrition*, 2004 Feb.; 79(2):261–7.

Savino, F., et al. *Lactobacillus reuteri* (American Type Culture Collection Strain 55730) versus simethicone in the treatment of infantile colic: a prospective randomized study. *Pediatrics*, 2007 Jan.; 119(1): e124–130.

Savino, F., et al. Intestinal microflora in breastfed colicky and non-colicky infants. *Acta Paediatrica*, 2004 June; 93(6):825–829.

Seppo, J., et al. Probiotics That Modify Disease Risk. *Journal of Nutrition*, May 2005; 135:1294–1298.

Szajewska, H. and Mrukowicz, J.Z. Use of probiotics in children with acute diarrhea. *Paediatric Drugs*, 2005; 7(2):111–122.

Weizman, A., et al. Effect of a probiotic infant formula on infections in child care centres: comparison of two probiotic agents. *Pediatrics*, 2005; 115:5–9.

CHAPTER 8

Bergonzelli, G.E., et al. Probiotics as a treatment strategy for gastro-intestinal diseases? *Digestion*, 2005; 72:57–68.

Bittner, A.C., et al. Prescript-assist probiotic-prebiotic treatment for irritable bowel syndrome: an open-label, partially controlled, 1-year extension of a previously published controlled clinical trial. *Clinical Therapy*, 2007; 29(6):1153–60.

Faber, S., et al. The use of probiotics in the treatment of irritable bowel syndrome: two case reports. *Alternative Therapies in Health and Medicine*, 2005; 11:60–62.

Goh, J., Morain, C. Review article: Nutrition and adult inflammatory bowel disease. *Alimentary Pharmacology and Therapeutics*, 2003; 17:307–320.

Gordon, L.V., et al. Epithelial cell growth and differentiation. III. Promoting diversity in the intestine: conversations between the microflora, epithelium, and diffuse GALT. *American Journal of Physiology*, 1997; 273:G565–G570.

Guslandi, M. Probiotics for chronic intestinal disorders. *American Journal of Gastroenterology*, 2003; 98:520–521.

Jonkers, D. and Stockbrügger, R. Probiotics and inflammatory bowel disease. *Journal of the Royal Society of Medicine*, 2003; 96:167–171.

Kanauchi, O., et al. Modification of intestinal flora in the treatment of inflammatory bowel disease. *Current Pharmaceutical Design*, 2003; 9:333–346.

Kanauchi, O., et al. The beneficial effects of microflora, especially obligate anaerobes, and their products on the colonic environment in inflammatory bowel disease. *Current Pharmaceutical Design*, 2005; 8(11)1047–1053.

Mahida, Y.R. and Rolfe, V.E. Host-bacterial interactions in inflammatory bowel disease. *Clinical Science*, 2004; 107:331–341.

Marteau, P., et al. Manipulation of the bacterial flora in inflammatory bowel disease. *Best Practice and Research Clinical Gastroenterology*, 2003; 17(1):47–61.

Marteau, P., et al. Probiotics and intestinal health effects: a clinical perspective. *British Journal of Nutrition*, 2002; 88(1):S51–S57.

Mimura, T., et al. Once daily high dose probitoic therapy (VSL#3) for maintaining remission in recurrent or refactory pouchitis. *Gut,* 2004; 53:108–114.

Niedzielin, K., et al. A controlled, double-blind, randomized study on the efficacy of Lactobacillus plantarum 299V in patients with irritable bowel syndrome. *European Journal of Gastroenterology and Hepatology,* 2001; 13:1143–1147.

Nobaek, S., et al. Alteration of intestinal microflora is associated with reduction in abdominal bloating and pain in patients with irritable bowel syndrome. *American Journal of Gastroenterology,* 2000; 13:1143–1147.

O'Mahony, L., et al. *Lactobacillus* and *Bifidobacterium* in irritable bowel syndrome: Symptom responses and relationship to cytokine profiles. *Gastroenterology,* 2005; 128:541–551.

Rath, H.C., et al. Differential Induction of Colitis and Gastritis in HLA-B27 Transgenic Rats Selectively Colonized with *Bacteroides vulgatus* or *Escherichia coli. Gastroenterology,* 1988; 114:519–526.

Seksik, P., et al. Review article: The role of bacteria in onset and perpetuation of inflammatory bowel disease. *Alimentary Pharmacology and Therapeutics,* 2006; 24(3):11–18.

Shanahan, F. Probiotics and inflammatory bowel disease: from fads and fantasy to facts and future. *British Journal of Nutrition,* 2002; 88(S1):S5–S9.

Shanahan, F. Probiotics and inflammatory bowel disease: is there a scientific rationale? *Inflammatory Bowel Diseases,* 2000; 6:107–115.

Shanahan, F. Probiotics in inflammatory bowel disease. *Gut,* 2001; 48:609.

Steidler, L., et al. Treatment of murine colitis by *Lactococcus lactis* secreting interleukin-10. *Science,* 2000; 289:1352–1355.

Szilagyi, A. Use of prebiotics for inflammatory bowel disease. *Canadian Journal of Gastroenterology,* 2005; 19(8):505–10.

Tomsen, M. Probiotics—enhancing health with beneficial bacteria. *Alternative Complementary Therapy,* 2006 Feb.:14–21.

Xavier, R.J. and D.K. Podolsky. How to get along—friendly microbes in a hostile world. *Science,* 2000; 289:1560–1563.

CHAPTER 9

Abrahamsson, T.R., et al. Probiotics in prevention of IgE-associated eczema: a double-blind, randomized, placebo-controlled trial. *Journal of Allergy and Clinical Immunology,* 2007; 119(5):1174–1180.

Barbeau, M. and H.L. Bpharm. Burden of atopic dermatitis in Canada. *International Journal of Dermatology,* 2006; 45(1):31–36.

Bongaerts, G.P. and Severijnen, R.S. Preventive and curative effects of probiotics in atopic patients. *Medical Hypotheses,* 2005; 64(6):1089–1092.

Boyle, R.J. and Tang, M.L.The role of probiotics in the management of allergic disease. *Clinical and Experimental Allergy,* 2006; 36(5):568–576.

Brouwer, M.L., et al. No effects of probiotics on atopic dermatitis in infancy: a randomized placebo controlled trial. *Clinical and Experimental Allergy,* 2006; 36(7):899–906.

Del Giudice, M.M., et al. Probiotics in the atopic march: highlights and new insights. *Digestive and Liver Disease,* 2006; 38(2):S288–290.

Forsythe, P., et al. Oral treatment with live probiotics may help alleviate allergic asthmatic response. *American Journal of Respiratory and Critical Care Medicine,* 2007; 175:561–569.

Furrie, E. Probiotics and allergy. *Proceedings of the Nutrition Society,* 2005; 64(4):465–469.

Holt, P., et al. A potential vaccine strategy for asthma and allied atopic diseases during early childhood. *Lancet,* 1994; 344:456–458.

Isolauri, E., et al. Probiotics in the management of atopic eczema. *Clinical and Experimental Allergy,* 2000; 30(11):1604–10.

Kalliomaki, M., et al. Probiotics and prevention of atopic disease: 4-year follow-up of a randomized placebo-controlled trial. *Lancet.* 2003; 361:1869–1871.

Kim, H., et al. Oral probiotic bacterial administration suppressed allergic responses in an ovalbumin-induced allergy mouse model. *Immunology and Medical Microbiology,* 2005; 45(4):259–67.

Kirjavainen, P., et al. Aberrant composition of gut microbiota of allergic infants: a target of bifidobacterial therapy at weaning? *Gut,* 2002; 51:51–55.

Kukkonen, K., et al. Probiotics and prebiotic galacto-oligosaccharides in the prevention of allergic diseases: A randomized, double-blind, placebo-controlled trial. *Journal of Allergy and Clinical Immunology*, 2007 Jan.; 119(1):192–8. E-publication 2006 Oct. 23.

Laitinen, K. and Isolarui, E. Management of food allergy: vitamins, fatty acids or probiotics? *European Journal of Gastroenterology and Hepatology*, 2005; 17(12):1305–11.

Majamaa, H. and Isolauri, E. Probiotics: A novel approach in the management of food allergy. *Journal of Allergy and Clinical Immunology*, 1997; 99:179–185.

Muñoz-López, F. Mucosae, allergy and probiotics. *Allergologia et immunopathologia*, 2004; 32:313–315.

Ouwehand, A., and Vesterlund, S. Health aspects of probiotics. *Investigational Drugs Journal*, 2003; 6(6):573–580.

Presentation: The Clinical and Immunological Effects of Early Probiotic Supplementation in Infants at High Risk of Allergic Disease: A Randomized, Controlled Trial. Abstract 161. Freiburger Allergy Prevention Study (FAPS): Effect of Lactobacillus GG on the Proliferative Response and Cytokine Levels in Isolated Mononuclear Cells of Mothers and Their Neonates. Abstract 162. Congress of the European Academy of Allergology and Clinical Immunology, June 10–14, 2006.

Rosenfeldt, V., et al. Effect of probiotic *Lactobacillus* strains in children with atopic dermatitis. *Journal of Allergy and Clinical Immunology*, 2003; 111:389–395.

Sistek, D., et al. Is the effect of probiotics on atopic dermatitis confined to food sensitized children? *Clinical and Experimental Allergy*, 2006; 36(5):629–33.

Tomsen, M. Probiotics—enhancing health with beneficial bacteria. *Alternative and Complementary Therapy*, Feb. 2006:14–21.

Vanderhoof, J.A. and Young, R. J. Probiotics in pediatrics. *Pediatrics*, 2002; 109:956–958.

Viljanen, M, et al. Probiotic effects of faecal inflammatory markers and on faecal IgA in food allgeric atopic eczema/dermatitis syndrome infants. *Pediatric Allergy and Immunology*, 2005; 16(1):65–71.

Weston S, et al. Effects of probiotics on atopic dermatitis: A randomized controlled trial. *Archives of Disease in Childhood*, 2005; 90:892–897.

CHAPTER 10

Leahy, S.C., et al. Getting better with *bifidobacteria*. *Journal of Applied Microbiology*, 2005; 98:1303–1315.

Levri, K.M., et al. Do probiotics reduce adult lactose intolerance? A systemic review. *Journal of Family Practice*, 2005; 54(7):613–20.

Lin, M.Y., et al. Management of lactose maldigestion by consuming milk containing *lactobacilli*. *Digestive Diseases and Sciences*, 1998; 43(1):133–137.

Marteau, P., et al. Probiotics and intestinal health effects: a clinical perspective. *British Journal of Nutrition*, 2002; 88(1):S51–S57.

Saltzman, J.R., et al. A randomized trial of *Lactobacillus acidophilus* BG2FO4 to treat lactose intolerance. *American Journal of Clinical Nutriton*, 1999; 69(1):140–6.

Vonk, R.J., et al. Lactose intolerance: analysis of underlying factors. *European Journal of Clinical Investigation*, 2003; 33(1):70–75.

Yesovitch, R., et al. Failure to improve parameters of lactose maldigestion using the multiprobiotic product VSL3 in lactose maldigesters: a pilot study. *Canadian Journal of Gastroenterology*, 2004; 18(2):83–86.

Zhong, Y., et al. Effect of probiotics and yogurt on colonic microflora in subjects with lactose intolerance. *Wei Sheng Yan Jiu*, 2006; 35(5):587–591.

Zhong, Y., et al. The role of colonic microbiota in lactose intolerance. *Digestive Disease Science*, 2004; 49(1):78–83.

CHAPTER 11

Aslim, B. and Kilic, E. Some probiotic properties of vaginal lactobacilli isolated from healthy women. *Japanese Journal of Infectious Disease*, 2006; 59(4):249–253.

Falagus, M.E., et al. Probiotics for prevention of recurrent urinary tract infections in women: a review of the evidence from microbiological and clinical studies. *Drugs*, 2006; 66(9):1253–1261.

Falagas, M.E., et al. Probiotics for prevention of recurrent vulvovaginal candidiasis: a review. *Journal of Antimicrobial Chemotherapy*, 2006; 58(2):266–272.

Korshunov, V.M., et al. The vaginal *Bifidobacterium* flora in women of reproductive age. *Zhurnal mikrobiologii, epidemiologii, i immunobiologii,* 1999; 4:74–78.

Marelli, G., et al. *Lactobacilli* for prevention of urogenital infections: a review. *European Review for Medical and Pharmacological Sciences,* 2004; 8(2):87–95.

McLean, N.M, and Rosenstein, I.J. Characterisation and selection of a *Lactobacillus* species to recolonise the vagina of women with recurrent bacterial vaginosis. *Journal of Medical Microbiology,* 2000; 49(6):543–552.

Reid, G. Could probiotics be an option for treating and preventing urogential infections? Medscape General Media, 2001; 3. Online document at www.medscape.com.viewarticle/408951. Accessed January 19, 2006.

Reid, G., et al. Probiotic *Lactobacillus* dose required to restore and maintain a normal vaginal flora. *FEMS Immunology and Medical Microbiology,* 2001; 132:37–41.

Reid, G., et al. Oral use of *Lactobacillus rhamnosus* GR-1 and *L. fermentum* RC-14 significantly alters vaginal flora: Randomized, placebo-controlled trial in 64 healthy women. *FEMS Immunology and Medical Microbiology,* 2003; 35:131–134.

Reid, G. Probiotic agents to protect the urogenitial tract against infection. *American Journal of Clinical Nutrition,* 2001; 73(2[suppl]):437S–443S.

Rousseau, V., et al. Prebiotic effects of oligosaccharides on selected vaginal *lactobacilli* and pathogenic microorganisms. *Anaerobe,* 2005; 11(3):145–153.

Tomsen, M. Probiotics—enhancing health with beneficial bacteria. *Alternative and Complementary Therapry,* Feb. 2006: 14–21.

Zarate, G. and Nader-Macias, M.E. Influence of probiotic vagainal *lactobacilli* on in vitro adhesion of urogenital pathogens to vaginal epithelial cells. *Letters in Applied Microbiology,* 2006; 43(2):174–180.

Zarate, G., et al. Protective effect of vaginal *Lactobacillis paracasei* CRL 1289 against urogenital infection produced by *Staphylococcus aureus* in a mouse animal mode. *Infectious Diseases in Obstetrics and Gynecology* 2007, Mar. 28; 48358 (e-publication).

CHAPTER 12

Devareddy, L., et al. The effects of fructo-oligosaccharides in combination with soy protein on bone in osteopenic ovariectomized rats. *Menopause*, 2006; 13(4):692–699.

Graci, S., DeMarco, C. and Rao, L. *The Bone-Building Solution*. Wiley; Mississauga, 2006.

Knapen, M.H.J., Schurgers, L.J., and Vermeer, C. Vitamin K2 supplementation improves hip bone geometry and bone strength indices in postmenopausal women. *Osteoporosis International*, 2007; Published online, 10.1007/s00198-007-0337-9.

Mutus, R., et al. The effect of dietary probiotic supplementation on tibial bone characteristics and strength in broilers. *Poultry Science*, 2006; 85(9):1621–1625.

Scholz-Ahrens, K.E., et al. Effects of prebiotics on mineral absorption. *American Journal of Clinical Nutrition*, 2001; 73(2):459S–464S.

Scholz-Ahrens, K.E., et al. Prebiotics, probiotics and synbiotics affect mineral absorption, bone mineral content and bone structure. *Journal of Nutrition*, 2007; 137(S2):838S–846S.

CHAPTER 13

Agerholm-Larsen, L., et al. The effect of a probiotic milk product on plasma cholesterol: A meta-analysis of short-term intervention studies. *European Journal of Clinical Nutrition*, 2000; 54:856–860.

Aihara, K., et al. Effect of powdered fermented milk with *Lactobacillus helveticus* on subjects with high-normal blood pressure or mild hypertension. *Journal of the American College of Nutrition*, 2005; 24(4):257–65.

De Smet, I., et al. Cholesterol lowering in pigs through enhanced bacterial bile salt hydrolase activity. *British Journal of Nutrition*, 998; 79:185–194.

Gill, H.S. and Guarner, F. Probiotics and human health: A clinical perspective. *Journal of Postgraduate Medicine*, 2004; 80:516–526.

Jauhiainen, T. and Korpela, R. Milk peptides and blood pressure. *Journal of Nutrition*, 2007; 137(3 Suppl 2):825S–9S.

Kiessling, G., et al. Long-term consumption of fermented dairy products over 6 months increases HDL cholesterol. *European Journal of Clinical Nutrition*, 2002; 56:843–849.

Klaver, F.A.M. and Van der Meer, R. The assumed assimilation of cholesterol by lactobacilli and *Bifidobacterium bifidum* is due to their bile salt-deconjugating activity. *Applied and Environmental Microbiology*, 1993; 59:1120–1124.

Liong, M. T. and Shah, N.P. Bile salt deconjugation ability, bile salt hydrolase activity and cholesterol co-precipitation ability of Lactobacilli strains. *International Dairy Journal* 2005; 15:391–398.

Liong, M.T. Probiotics: a critical review of their potential role as antihypertensives, immune modulators, hypocholesterolemics, and perimenopausal treatments. *Nutrition Reviews*, 2007; 65(7):316–28.

Moser, S.A. and Savage, D.C. Bile salt hydrolase activity and resistance to toxicity of conjugated bile salts are unrelated properties in *lactobacilli*. *Applied and Environmental Microbiology*, 2001; 67(8):3476–3480.

Murray, B.A. and R.J. FitzGerald. Angiotensin converting enzyme inhibitory peptides derived from food proteins: biochemistry, bioactivity and production. *Current Pharmaceutical Design*, 2007; 13(8):773–91.

Naruszewicz, M., et al. Effect of *Lactobacillus plantarum* 299v on cardiovascular disease risk factors in smokers. *American Journal of Clinical Nutrition*, 2002; 76:1249–1255.

Pereira, D.I. and Gibson, G.R. Effects of consumption of probiotics and prebiotics on serum lipid levels in humans. *Critical Reviews in Biochemistry and Molecular Biology*, 2002; 37:259–281.

Sarkar, S. Potential of acidophilus milk to lower cholesterol. *Nutrition and Food Science*, 2003; 33(6):273–277.

St-Onge, M.P., et al. Consumption of fermented and nonfermented dairy products: effects on cholesterol concentrations and metabolism. *American Journal of Clinical Nutrition*, 2000; 71:674–681.

Tanaka, H., et al. Screening of lactic acid bacteria for bile salt hydrolase activity. *Journal of Dairy Science*, 1999; 82:2530–2535.

Tomsen, M. Probiotics—enhancing health with beneficial bacteria. *Journal of Alternative and Complementary Medicine*, 2006 Feb.: 14–21.

Chapter 14

Benno, Y., et al. Human fecal flora in health and colon cancer. *Acta chirurgica Scandinavica*, 1991; S562:15–23.

Bergonzelli, G.E., et al. Probiotics as a treatment strategy for gastrointestinal diseases? *Digestion*, 2005; 72:57–68.

Boutron, M.C., et al. Calcium, phosphorus, vitamin D, dairy products and colorectal carcinogenesis: a French case-control study. *British Journal of Cancer*, 1996; 74:145–151.

Budagov, R.S., et al. The protective activity of a new variant of the probiotic Acilact in exposure to ionizing radiation and anticancer chemotherapy under experimental conditions. *Vestnik Rossiĭskoĭ Akademii Meditsinskikh Nauk*, 2006; (2):3–5.

Coakley, M., et al. Conjugated linoleic acid biosynthesis by human-derived *Bifidobacterium* species, *Journal of Applied Microbiology*, 2003; 94:138–145.

Delia, P., et al. Use of probiotics for prevention of radiation-induced diarrhea. *World Journal of Gastroenterology*, 2007 February; 13(6):912–915.

El-Nezami, H.S., et al. Probiotic supplementation reduces a biomarker for increased risk of liver cancer in young men from Southern China. *American Journal of Clinical Nutrition*, 2006; 83:1199–1203.

Leahy, S.C., et al. Getting better with bifidobacteria. *Journal of Applied Microbiology*, 2004; 98:1303–1305.

Pool-Zobel, B.L., et al. *Lactobacillus* and *Bifidobacterium*-mediated antigenotoxicity in the colon of rats. *Nutrition and Cancer*, 1996; 26:365–380.

Rafter, J. The effects of probiotics on colon cancer development. *Nutrition Research Reviews*, 2004; 17:277–284.

Rosberg-Cody, E., et al. Mining the microbiota of the neonatal gastrointestinal tract for conjugated linoleic acid-producing bifidobacteria. *Applied and Environmental Microbiology*, 2004; 70:4635–4641.

Rowland, I.R., et al. Effect of *Bifidobacterium longum* and inulin on gut bacteria metabolism and carcinogen-induced aberrant crypt foci in rats. *Carcinogenesis*, 1998; 19:281–285.

Tavan, E., et al. Antimutagenic activities of various lactic acid bacteria against food mutagens: heterocyclic amines. *Journal of Dairy Research*, 2002; 69:335–341.

Wollowski, I., et al. Protective role of probitocs and prebiotics in colon cancer. *American Journal of Clinical Nutrition*, 2001; 73:S451–S455.

CHAPTER 15

Bergonzelli, G.E., et al. Probiotics as a treatment strategy for gastrointestinal diseases? *Digestion* 2005; 72:57–68.

Lam, E.K., et al. Probiotic *Lactobacillus rhamnosus* GG enhances gastric ulcer healing in rats. *European Journal of Pharmacology*, 2007; 565(1–3):171–179.

Marteau, P., et al. Probiotics and intestinal health effects: a clinical perspective. *British Journal of Nutrition*, 2002; 88(1):S51–S57.

Saggioro, A., et al. *Helicobacter pylori* eradication with *Lactobacillus reuteri*. A double-blind placebo-controlled study. *Journal of Digestive and Liver Disease*, 2005; 37(1): S88.

Tomsen, Michael. Probiotics—enhancing health with beneficial bacteria. *Alternative and Complementary Therapy*, 2006 Feb.: 14–21.

Unknown. *L. reuteri* supplement reduces side effects of H. pylori eradication therapy in children. *Nature Clinical Practice Gastroenterology and Hepatology*, 2007; 4, 66–67.

Wang, K.Y., et al. Effects of ingesting *Lactobacillus* and *Bifidobacterium*-containing yogurt in subjects with colonized *Helicobacter pylori*. *American Journal of Clinical Nutrition*, 2004; 80:737–741.

CHAPTER 16

Ahola, A.J., et al. Short-term consumption of probiotic-containing cheese and its effect on dental caries risk factors. *Archives of Oral Biology*, 2002; 47: 799–804.

Brudnak, M.A. Application of genomeceuticals to the molecular and immunological aspects of autism. *Medical Hypotheses*, 2001; 57(2):186–91.

Castagliulo, I., et. al. *S. boulardii* protease inhibits effects of *C. difficile* toxins A and B in human colonic mucosa. *Infection and Immunity,* 1999; 67:302–7.

Clayton, J. Friendly bacteria to fight HIV. *Lancet,* 2002; 2:392.

de Vrese, M., et al. Effect of *Lactobacillus gasseri* PA 16/8, *Bifidobacterium longum* SP07/3, *B. bifidum* MF20/5 on common cold episodes: a double blind, randomized, controlled trial. *Clinical Nutrition,* 2005; 24(4):481–490.

de Vrese, M., et al. Probiotic bacteria reduced duration and severity but not the incidence of common cold episodes in a double blind, randomized, controlled trial. *Vaccine,* 2006 10; 24(44–46):6670–6674.

d'Souza, A.L., et al. Probiotics in prevention of antibiotic associated diarrhea: meta-analysis. *British Medical Journal,* 2002; 324.

Ewaschuk, J., et al. Probiotic bacteria prevent hepatic damage and maintain colonic barrier function in a mouse model of sepsis. *Hepatology,* 2007; 46(3):841–50.

Gaon, D., et al. Lactose digestion by milk fermented with human strains of *Lactobacillus acidophilus* and *Lactobacillus casei. Medicina* (Buenos Aires), 1995; 55:237–242.

Gorbach, et al. Successful treatment of relapsing *C. difficile* colitis with *Lactobacillus* GG. *Lancet,* 1987; ii:1519.

Hatakka, K., et al. Probioitcs reduce the prevalence of oral *candida* in the elderly—a randomized controlled trial. *Journal of Dental Research,* 2007; 86(2):125–130.

Hove, H., Nordgaard-Andersen, I., Mortensen, P.B. Effect of lactic acid bacteria on the intestinal production of lactate and short-chain fatty acids, and the absorption of lactose. *American Journal of Clinical Nutrition,* 1994 Jan.; 59(1):74–9.

Ibrahim, F., et al. Probiotic bacteria as potential detoxification tools: assessing their heavy metal binding isotherms. *Can J Microbiol,* 2006; 52(9):877–85.

Johnston, B.J. and Vohra, S. Treating C. difficile. *Canadian Medical Association Journal,* 2005; 172(4).

Lahtinen, S.J., et al. Specific *Bifidobacterium* strains isolated from elderly subjects inhibit growth of *Staphylococcus aureus. International Journal of Food Microbiology.* 2007; 177(1):125–128.

Lewis, S., et al. Effect of the prebiotic oligofructose on relapse of *Clostridium difficile*-associated diarrhea: a randomized, controlled study. *Clinical Gastroenterology and Hepatology*, 2005; 3(5):442–8.

Marteau P, et al. Probiotics and intestinal health effects: a clinical perspective. *British Journal of Nutrition* 2002; 88(1):S51–S57.

Miyazaki, K., et al. *Bifidobacterium*-fermented soy milk extract stimulates hylauronic acid production in human skin cells and hairless mouse skin. *Skin Pharmacology and Applied Skin Physiology*, 2003; 16(3):108–116.

Miyazaki, K.,et al. Topical application of *Bifidobacterium*-fermented soy milk extract containing genistein and daidzein improves rheological and physiological properties of skin. *Journal of Cosmetic Science*, 2004; 55(5):473–479.

Naaber, P., et al. Inhibition of *Clostridium difficile* strains by intestinal *Lactobacillus* species. *Journal of Medical Microbiology*, 2004; 53:551–554.

Nase, L., et al. Effect of long-term consumption of a probiotic bacterium, *Lactobacillus rhamnosus* GG, in milk on dental caries and caries risk in children. *Caries Research*, 2001; 35: 412–420.

Park, S.H., et al. Effects of occupational metallic mercury vapor exposure on suppressor-inducer (CD4+CD45RA+) T lymphocytes and CD57+CD16+ natural killer cells. *International Archives of Occupational and Environmental Health*, 2000; 73(8):537–42.

Plummer, S., et al. *Clostridium difficile* pilot study: effects of probiotic supplementation on the incidence of C. *difficile* diarrhoea. *Internal Microbiology*, 2004; 7(1):59–62.

Pochapin, M. The effect of probiotics on *Clostridium difficile* diarrhea. *American Journal of Gastroenterology*, 2000; 95(1):S11–S13.

Sokhee, S., et al. Lactic acid bacteria from healthy oral cavity of Thai volunteers: inhibition of oral pathogens. *Journal of Applied Microbiology*, 2001; 90:172–179.

Worth, R.G., et al. Mercury inhibition of neutrophil activity: evidence of aberrant cellular signaling and incoherent cellular metabolism. *Scandinavian Journal of Immunology*, 2001; 53(1):49–55.

CHAPTER 17

Boyle, R.J., et al. Probiotic use in clinical practice: what are the risks? *American Journal of Clinical Nutrition*, 2006; 83(6):1256–1264.

Ezendam, J. and van Loveren, H. Probiotics: immunomodulation and evaluation of safety and efficacy. *Nutrition Review*, 2006; 64(1):1–14.

Land, M.H., et al. *Lactobacillus* sepsis associated with probiotic therapy. *Pediatrics*, 2005; 115(1):178–181.

Land, M.H., et al. *Lactobacillus* sepsis associated with probiotic therapy. *Pediatrics* 2005; 116(2):517.

Salminen, M.K., et al. *Lactobacillus* bacteremia, clinical significance and patient outcome, with special focus on probiotic *L. rhamnosus* GG. *Clinical Infectious Diseases*, 2004; 38:62–68.

Salminen, S., et al. Demonstration of safety of probiotics—a review. *International Journal of Food Microbiology*, 1998; 44(1–2):93–106.

Index

About the Author

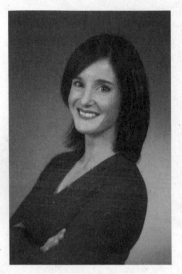

Allison Tannis B.Sc., M.Sc., RHN is a leading nutritional scientist and educator, and a Registered Holistic Nutritionist. She is the author of *Vitality: Quest for a healthy diet* as well as a writer for many health and nutrition publications across the country. Allison is the host of the radio feature *Healthy Living*.